"LOSING WEIGHT HAS NOTHING TO DO WITH GUESSING GAMES!"

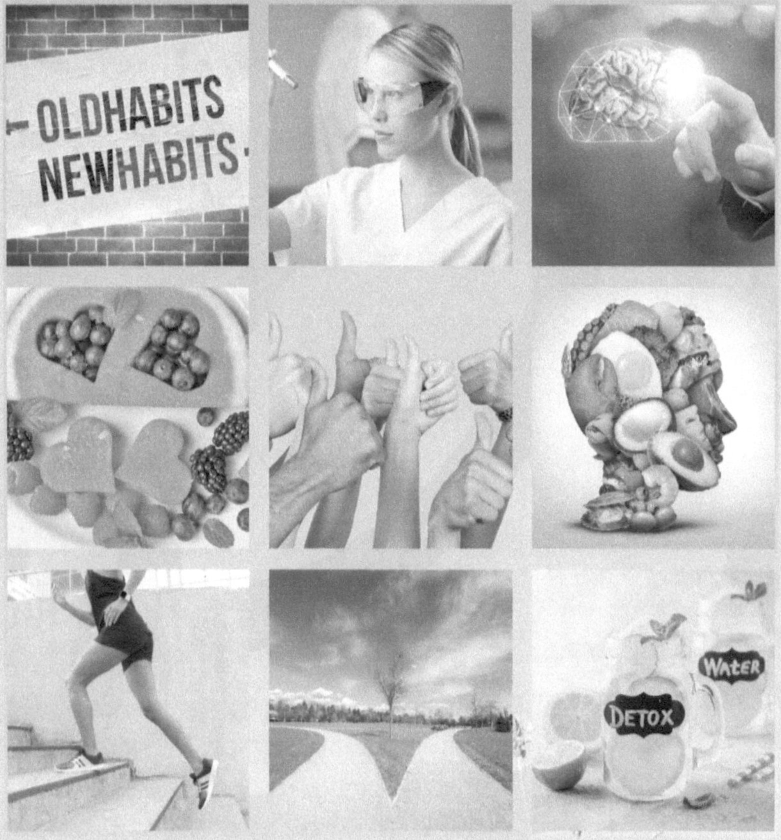

SMALL STEP HABITS CREATE WEIGHT LOSS SUCCESS

BASIC APPROACH IN DIETING. FORM NEW HABITS.. CHANGE YOUR LIFESTYLE WITHOUT SUFFERING

like putty. You raise your arms, and the muscle looks like they're sitting on the wrong end. Whether it took you forty pounds to notice the weight gain, or you gasped when you saw five pounds extra on the scale this morning, you require some help.

Being overweight doesn't only steal from your health like a thief in the night. It sends you on an emotional rollercoaster of crash diets and starvation. You've probably tried twenty diets and listened to every piece of advice from doctors who've told you to lose weight before your health takes another dip, but it doesn't matter how hard you've tried, you still can't shake the pounds. Moreover, you've popped miracle cures for weight loss like candy, and nothing has changed.

You feel worse after all the failed journeys. Don't worry if you're new to the weight loss pursuit, either. You'll learn that the word "diet" is the enemy unless you understand how you can change your lifestyle and shed those pounds, burn that fat, and tone up for the beach. The media promote diets, the very people who get paid to sell miracle cures for weight loss. Diets are anything but good. Weight loss is a journey you must take, and every tiny step you reach will bring you closer to the outcome, whether the outcome is a stream-lined body or to fit back into your favorite shirt.

The media makes you feel like you can't do it unless you buy every product, sign up for every membership, and work with a paid coach who pays for advertising on media channels. If the diets work, why are the statistics telling a different tale? Do you know how the media promotes the products through subliminal messages other than direct sales pitches? Every advertisement you can think of is promoting healthier lifestyles, skinnier bodies, and model physiques.

Travel adverts show slender women lying on the beach. They show ruggedly handsome men with six-packs that seem

INTRODUCTION

Jim Rohn once said, "Take care of your body. It's the only place you have to live." Your body is the home you'll have for the rest of your life. Sometimes, it might be a little stuffed, popping with a few extra pounds hanging from the windows. For some, the seams are about to burst, and it's only a matter of time before the home is filled with unwanted health issues and missed opportunities.

How often have you visited a doctor over the last few years? How much money have you wasted on diet plans, nutritional changes, and medication that only stops you from losing weight? How many diagnoses have you had to endure throughout your gradual weight gain? Diabetes, heart disorders, depression, anxiety, blood pressure issues, cholesterol, and even chronic fatigue are on the cards when you carry extra weight.

How many of these conditions have you had to face? How many more do you still want to endure? Weight gain might look like it pops up overnight. You were so skinny just a few months ago, but now you can play with the new flab around your waist

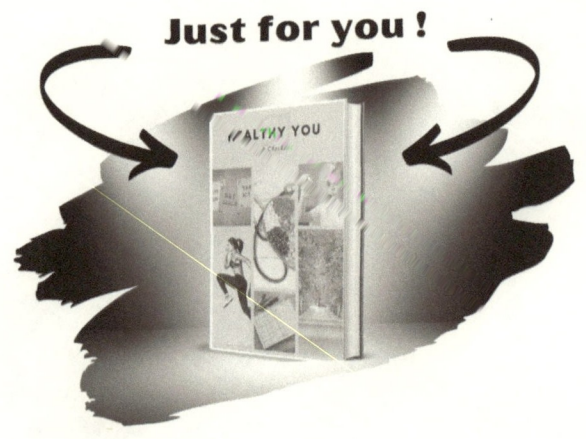

A Special Gift to our Readers

Included with your purchases out Task Checklist Guide to help you on your journey. This step-by-step task guide will prepare you in getting the correct steps in getting healthy.

Click the link below and let us know which email address to send it too.

Healthy You - Task Checklist

www.amazingjaqproducts.com/publishing/HealthyYou

The Keto Lifestyle	52
The Value of Sleep	55
STEP SIX: BREAKING AWAY FROM THE FORK IN THE ROAD... THE PLATEAU	57
Standing Your Ground	57
Hitting the Plateau	59
Quick Fix for Breaking the Plateau	62
STEP SEVEN: TREAT YOURSELF DESERVEDLY	65
Hijacking the Reward Loop	65
Climbing the SMART Ladder	67
Rewarding Each Rung	69
Afterword	73
Plee From Author	77
References	79

CONTENTS

Just For You — vii
Introduction — ix

HOW OUR BEHAVIOR WORKS — 1
False Perceptions — 1
The Faster, the Better — 5
Breaking Through the Myths — 8

STEP ONE: REMOVE THE DOUBTFUL MINDSET — 9
What Self-Doubt Does to You — 9
Learning About Cause and Effect — 12
Shifting Your Mindset for Optimal Results — 13
The 21-Day Confidence Boost — 16

STEP TWO: UNDERSTAND YOUR BODY WITH THE RIGHT TESTS — 19
Why Test? — 19
Functional Tests to Consider — 21

STEP THREE: ADDING NUTRITION AND FOOD STRATEGIES — 27
What Does Clean Eating Mean? — 27
How to Eat Clean — 29

STEP FOUR: MASTERING THE HABIT OF BEING FIT — 37
The 30-Day Challenge — 37
10-Minute Workouts — 40
Endless Possibilities — 45

STEP FIVE: ADDING A FEW CELLULAR CHOICES — 47
Detoxing Your Body — 47
Intermittent Fasting for Weight Loss — 50

COPYRIGHT

© Copyright 2020 by Amazing JAQ Products, LLC - All rights reserved.

The content contained within this book may not be reproduced, duplicated or transmitted without direct written permission from the author or the publisher.

Under no circumstances will any blame or legal responsibility be held against the publisher, or author, for any damages, reparation, or monetary loss due to the information contained within this book, either directly or indirectly.

Legal Notice:

This book is copyright protected. It is only for personal use. You cannot amend, distribute, sell, use, quote or paraphrase any part, or the content within this book, without the consent of the author or publisher.

Disclaimer Notice:

Please note the information contained within this document is for educational and entertainment purposes only. All effort has been executed to present accurate, up to date, reliable, complete information. No warranties of any kind are declared or implied. Readers acknowledge that the author is not engaged in the rendering of legal, financial, medical or professional advice. The content within this book has been derived from various sources. Please consult a licensed professional before attempting any techniques outlined in this book.

By reading this document, the reader agrees that under no circumstances is the author responsible for any losses, direct or indirect, that are incurred as a result of the use of the information contained within this document, including, but not limited to, errors, omissions, or inaccuracies.

SMALL STEP HABITS CREATE WEIGHT LOSS SUCCESS

BASIC APPROACH IN DIETING. FORM NEW HABITS. CHANGE YOUR LIFESTYLE WITHOUT SUFFERING

PURE SMART LIFE

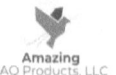

to have a life of their own under every business suit on television. You're being fed with constant ideas of what you must look like, each one making you feel even worse. The only benefit of subliminal ideations of perfect bodies is that it inspires you. The United States doesn't look like this in real life, and you're surrounded by people who follow every diet trend as you do.

More than 32% of US adults over the age of twenty were classified as obese in 2018. Obesity double-whammies us because we lose our primal health, making us suffer from diabetes and other chronic conditions, and it strips us of our longevity. Moreover, 28.5% of elderly Americans were obese by 2019. Their bodies are already declining, and being obese certainly doesn't make them live longer and enjoy their families and grandchildren.

The cost of medical bills due to obesity in the late 1990s was averaging $75 billion, but it increased to $147 billion annually by 2008. Understandably, not everyone who's trying to lose weight is obese either. Some people try to shed some pounds before they lose control of their weight. Weight-loss attempts saw 56.4% of women and 41.7% of men try fad diets and starvation exercises by 2016 (Drah, 2020). If these diet trends worked, wouldn't the country be slender, healthy, and toned?

Numbers don't lie, and they show you how trending diets haven't worked. Your body was never built for this yo-yo lifestyle. If only you knew that you could change your weight without weighing food, spending your life savings, and measuring every ounce you eat. No one ever told you that you could do this without the personal trainer that costs your retirement fund and the coach that makes you measure your waist every damn Monday morning.

You have the same goal as everyone battling these trending failures, except you can learn how to switch your body into a natural fat-burner and toner. Your body can do far more than you can believe. Your weight can drop with minor changes. You don't have to sell your soul to the devil or consume enough modern medicine to make your body maintain the weight. You need selfless assistance from someone who has your best interests at heart. You need guidance from someone who expects nothing in return.

How can you control the biology of your body without knowing how it works and how everything you consume is loaded with chemicals and toxins that prevent weight loss? You'll understand what the food industry is doing to you. You'll also learn why these fad diets aren't working and how you can make small changes and still get huge results. It starts in the mind, so you'll learn how to set your mind for the changes to come. You'll learn about the tests that help you design a lifestyle where diets aren't needed.

I'll teach you how to eat clean and still enjoy the favorites you've previously abstained from. The world has a twisted idea of weight loss, and who knew that making such small changes to your daily eating habits could bring such rewards? There will be workouts you can use to enhance your journey and tighten that butt. Tone your abs and target specific problem areas to shed those stubborn pounds with practical ten-minute workouts. Exercise is enjoyable when you know how to master what you need.

You'll also learn about four proven methods of turning your body's natural biology into an unstoppable fat-burning monster. I've even thrown in some simple charts to help you use the techniques that promote weight loss and better health in the long-term. You'll know where things can seem insurmountable and how to overcome them with ease.

I've always had optimal health in mind because I want to be around for my kids until they grow old and grey. Maintaining a healthy weight has only been part of it. My entire family leads a healthy lifestyle, keeping weight down, and having the energy and happiness to enjoy every moment of life. Don't misunderstand me. I've had obstacles that hit me like a bat, but my family always overcame them. My daughter was the one to inspire my passion for ultimate health and tone that started a 10-year journey of research to understand every aspect of it.

Her chronic condition pulled every heartstring until I spent fifteen years researching, applying, and enjoying small changes that opened our lives to massive improvements. I wanted to be healthier, toned, and sustain an optimal body mass index (BMI) so that I could enjoy life with my family. We're highly active today, and it's all thanks to the small habits we changed over time. You don't need to rip the bandaid off because the picture-perfect person you desire is a long-term goal.

It starts when you throw away all the ideas you've had until now. Burn every miracle pill and unsubscribe from every magazine that makes you feel obsolete. My journey, experience, and advice will be natural so that you can return your body to the state it once was. Your body's ability to master health and weight is merely one small step ahead. All you must do is take the first one.

HOW OUR BEHAVIOR WORKS

Chapter 1

The problem with yo-yo diets, fad diets that make your weight rapidly fluctuate, isn't only that your weight goes up and down. Your moods, behavior, and happiness also fluctuate, leaving you with depression, misery, poor health, and regret. This form of dieting is even worse when you think you're eating right, but you're still avoiding the scale because it feels like a vendetta against you. You throw it in a locked closet, avoid mirrors, and pop miracle diet pills like it's going out of fashion, but is this really the life you want to live, or do you want to change it? It's time to learn about what's going on in the so-called healthy foods you've probably tried already. You'll learn about the most common myths in weight loss too.

False Perceptions

Your idea of healthy eating could be fueled by magazines, adverts, and billboards. What is the most common thing you see among these subliminal messages you're fed daily? Fruit and vegetables are the healthiest things you can eat, right? Clear your mind and let me explain why this isn't the *whole* truth. Over the ages, the world's population has exploded, and the food industry must keep up with the demand. Food is no longer simple as it once was, even fruit, vegetables, grains, rice, and wheat products. Everything we eat is laced with chemicals to speed the harvest up and to make the food last longer. It's unnatural that our foods are evolving into harmful products.

The first myth you must break is the one that commercially tells you what is healthy to eat. Pesticides and overly processed foods are stripping you of your success in healthy living and losing weight. Worst of all is that the taste of our food has improved, but this isn't for your benefit. It's for the benefit of the competing food industries. The first problem with modern food is that our fruit, vegetables, wheat, barley, oats, and everything in our agriculture are laced with pesticides. The most famous of them is called Monsanto Roundup. This product is used on everything, everywhere, but it has a killer ingredient, and I don't mean the good kind.

Roundup contains heavy amounts of glyphosate, a toxic chemical used to alter and eradicate the bacteria in the grains' structure. Remember that grains and anything that grows are living beings. The food industry can try to convince you that the residue left behind on our food is harmless, but the fact is that the human body also has a pathway running through it, connecting to the brain, gut, immune system, and every organ. This pathway is made up of bacteria that travels throughout the body when it's needed elsewhere. Humans have the same biological structure as plants when it comes to bacterial physiology.

Our gut is made of billions of good bacteria, and the Roundup residue *kills* it. Unfortunately, this bacterium is necessary for your ultimate health because all diseases, including obesity, start in the stomach. It isn't just the food you eat. It's also the chemicals you're exposed to, the additives that are thrown into your food to make it shinier and tastier, and it's the artificial flavors and colors that set our bacterium off balance. Obesity is a disease that leads to many other diseases. The chances are that you aren't obese if you've at least been trying to maintain a healthy weight, but any unnecessary weight affects you somehow.

Glyphosate damages the metabolism in your body, which is responsible for how your body processes food (Living Young, n.d.). It's sprayed on the wheat crops to dry it out faster for quicker harvesting. The highest numbers of this chemical are found in wheat, barley, and oats, but the residue is also found on fruits and vegetables, which are the very ingredients you've been told to eat to lose weight. These high-chemical grains appear in the store shortly after harvesting them as bread, bagels, and muffins, but the residue remains. Potatoes, peas, sugar beets, and corn also contain too much residue. Glyphosate disrupts the bacterium in the gut leading to many health problems other than weight gain.

Gut bacteria play a huge role in the immune system and other bodily functions. When good bacteria fall, harmful bacteria or pathogens take over, and they turn toxic. Your toxicity levels rise, and the immune system attacks these pathogens, causing inflammation. Chronic inflammation leads to allergies, cardiovascular problems, obesity, irritable bowel syndrome (IBS), and even depression. You can't lose weight if you're eating the wrong foods. Your food is also highly processed to make it more appealing than the competitors in the market. Apples never used to be so red and shiny. Now, they look like the apple that put Snow White in a coma.

Processed food might look and taste better, but it's packed to the brim with salt, sugar, and unhealthy fats. Processed food is anything that's been processed, packaged, altered, or refined. Unprocessed and natural foods are those that list one ingredient on the label. When you buy apples, make sure the only ingredient *is* apples. Otherwise, it has artificial enhancers and flavors. The human body wasn't made to contend with unnatural foods. Obviously, butter is processed before it comes to you, but margarine is a death trap of weight gain. Extra virgin olive oil is as natural as it comes up to the bottling process, but sunflower oil is hydrogenated, meaning that it was previously solidified to make it last longer. Hydrogenation only creates bad cholesterol with trans fats.

Refined sugar and high-fructose corn syrup contain enough empty calories to make you crave more sugar. It causes fat storage in the liver and abdomen, slowing down the metabolism. Bad cholesterol and insulin resistance are also on the cards with refined sugars. Artificial additives don't only make food more attractive, but they also preserve the products to last eons. The problem with artificial additives is that companies don't need to disclose their secret recipes, so you don't have a clue what you're eating. Aspartame is a substitute for sugar in sodas, and it promotes weight gain as it unbalances the bacterium in your stomach.

Refined carbohydrates are also dangerous because they turn into simple carbs that are digested so fast that you stay hungry. They don't satisfy you enough and break down too fast, leaving you craving more carbs. Processed food also loses its natural fiber, leading to constipation and a halted metabolism. The food industry claims to replace nutrients and vitamins lost in processed food, but they can't replace the natural substances. Worst of all, many of these ingredients listed on your processed foods are addictive. Companies must hook you to their foods and secret recipes somehow. So, the ingredients in these foods trigger addictive responses in the brain.

Dopamine is released, and this is a chemical from the brain that makes you feel happy. Don't be fooled by the "healthy products" adverts sell to you. Those adverts are paid for by companies that provide the foods. Only whole, natural, and clean foods are good for weight loss.

The Faster, the Better

Another common myth of weight loss is that we can use crash diets to lose weight fast. The reason this myth is blown up straight away is that losing weight is only half the challenge. You must maintain the weight loss to be successful with your new figure. The secret to dropping pounds, burning fat, and keeping it off is to do it slowly. Your body goes through a change, and no change has ever happened overnight. You didn't gain weight overnight, did you? Sadly, most crash dieters regain all the weight in the years that follow. The slower you lose weight, the longer you're likely to keep it off. Endocrinologist and obesity specialist Marcio Griebeler explains that everyone has a weight set-point (Cleveland Clinic, 2019).

Griebeler states that 80 to 95% of weight losers regain everything they've lost, and the culprit is the set-point in your body. Our weight set-point is made of various factors, including genetics, lifestyle, hormones, environments, and behavior. Your set-point works with your metabolism. This explains why weight gain is also gradual. Your body has a weight point that it loves resetting too. However, crash diets aren't going to alter the set-point. Only slow and steady diets can do this. There are too many biological fluctuations happening in your body when you enter a crash diet. Firstly, the body's set-point will simply readjust to the new calorie intake quickly, meaning that it won't be long before it can function as it normally does with fewer calories.

Suddenly, you need to eat even fewer calories to keep losing weight because the body has adapted now. The hormonal adjustment will drive you insane. Your levels of leptin decrease. This is the hormone that makes you feel full. Your levels of ghrelin will escalate, and this is the hormone that makes you feel hungry. The body knows how to preserve itself, and it will send your hormones into war to prevent starvation while it adjusts to the new calories. Your mind will also start playing tricks on you because everything will look and smell divine. The brain will crave unhealthy foods. Eating fewer calories will wreak havoc on your brain functions. The problem is that the effects last longer than the crash diet does.

Your body's retaliation doesn't stop with the hormones either. Do you want to lose weight, or are you planning to lose muscle mass? Crash diets aren't picky about what they take. Eating less than 500 calories daily will force the body to burn something for energy, and once the calories, carbs, and fats have burned, the body turns to the muscles. Crash diets often require you to measure your calories and eat less than what a child could survive on. This isn't the way to lose weight because you need muscles. Keep in mind that the metabolism also slows down because its function is determined by the number of calories it burns daily. Giving it no calories to burn is like starving it to learn how slow it must actually work.

Remember that your metabolism is going to adapt to new functions with a diet. Spending too much time on a fast crash diet, intended to lose weight rapidly, is going to train the metabolism to run slower for a long time. Now, you understand why you start gaining weight after the crash diet again. The metabolism can't keep up with the calories you eat after you stop dieting. The hormones that need to ignite the metabolism's work become scarce, such as the thyroid hormone. Crash diets can also lead to nutritional deficiencies that only make matters worse (Raman, 2017). Nutrients like iron, folate, and vitamin B 12 are missing, leading to a problem in various parts of your body while you're on this diet.

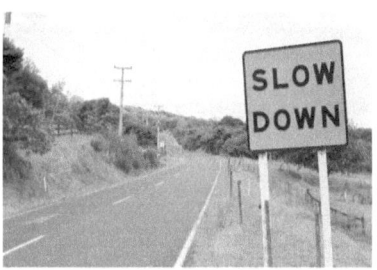

Slow and Steady

Eating too few calories makes you lose hair because there aren't enough nutrients to sustain hair growth. You won't be consuming enough vitamin D, phosphorus, and calcium to strengthen your bones anymore either. A lack of vital nutrients makes you tired as well, leading to extreme exhaustion and sometimes anemia. Anemia starts when your red blood cells, responsible for immune functions, are too depleted. Failing to consume the nutrients you need will only cause your immune system to falter, and you'll be more prone to infections and diseases. Mood swings, cold shivers, fatigue, muscle cramps, dizziness, and dehydration are more symptoms you can suffer from when you eat too few calories.

You might also develop gallstones which are rock-hard collections of digestive juices that sit too long in the gallbladder. Gallstones are painful, and they'll make your weight loss journey anything but pleasant. So, this myth is broken because the right amount of weight to lose weekly is between one and two pounds. You can't starve yourself either because your body won't allow it. You'll only be hurting yourself.

Breaking Through the Myths

Losing weight too fast is no way to maintain it after you've shed the weight. So, focus on leading a healthy lifestyle and forget about these diets that promise you ten pounds lost per week. Also, stay away from any diet products that make these promises too. Those products contain just as many harmful chemicals as the food you eat. Lose weight slowly because this is a marathon; it's not a race. It takes a life-long commitment to lower your metabolic set-point permanently. It's also advised to have a nutritional therapist on board. Speak to a functional medicine practitioner to also help you with natural supplements without consuming all the ingredients that could make weight loss impossible.

The first myth must also be broken, smashed, and tossed out of the highest skyscraper. You need to eat foods that contain the natural nutrients that supplement your weight loss desire. You can't eat these foods processed fifty times, sprayed with chemicals, pumped with additives, and still expect your metabolism to work correctly. Your body needs wholesome, natural, organic, and chemical-free produce straight from the farm. You should never buy anything with a long list of ingredients you can't even pronounce. Losing weight has nothing to do with diets.

It has everything to do with a change of lifestyle and adopting healthy habits which include eating whole foods, staying hydrated, exercising, and feeding your body with nutrients to promote weight loss. Forget about the word "diet" and start thinking about the rest of your life. Portion control, watching your intake, and losing weight slowly is how you happily get to the end of the marathon.

STEP ONE: REMOVE THE DOUBTFUL MINDSET

Chapter 2

Once you know what prevents you from losing weight in your daily diet, the first obstacle standing in your way is your mindset. It's easier to doubt yourself, feel uncertain, and be disappointed than it is to compliment yourself for a job well done. People find it near impossible to recognize what they've achieved, what they're capable of doing, and how small changes can make a big difference. It's part of human nature to doubt yourself, but you don't need to if you change your mindset.

What Self-Doubt Does to You

Self-doubt appears whenever we lack confidence in our abilities. You might think you don't have what it takes to reach your dream physique. We aren't good, strong, disciplined, or skilled enough to reach for our dreams and desires. I bet your deepest desire is to shed some pounds and lead a healthier lifestyle where happiness is bountiful. Be honest with yourself, do you feel like you can achieve this without a sliver of doubt creeping up on you? The fear of failure is the definition of doubt. A hint of doubt hasn't harmed anyone. It shows that you acknowledge what needs to be done to reach your dream, understanding what your current skills and knowledge gives you, and accepting that it needs some improvement.

You're reading this book, which means that you've doubted your weight loss abilities to some extent. That's the hint of doubt that's good for anyone, but self-doubt can become debilitating, causing you to fail before you start. Doubt works in cycles. Self-doubt happens so often, and we don't even realize it. Take an example of where a friend asks you how you lost five pounds. Your weight loss has staggered since, and now you tell your friend that your method didn't work. The fact is that it *did* work, and that's how you initially lost five pounds. You doubt yourself because of a past mistake. You were following the rules and you thought you were eating right. However, your weight loss still hit a brick wall.

Self-doubt started surfacing because you blame yourself for the failure. Do you think your friend would ask you how you did it if you failed in their eyes? Sometimes, your expectations are based on factors out of your control or they're set way too high. You expect yourself to be perfect, and you expect yourself to lose twenty pounds in two months as another friend did. Wait for it; they'll regain the weight soon enough. Self-doubt is born on the premise of many reasons. Past mistakes and experiences are obvious reasons why you think you'll fail again. Not every hat fits every change of clothes, and you shouldn't think that a previous failure guarantees another one. You didn't know enough last time, and you listened to all the paid adverts the food industry supplied for their convenience.

Mistakes of any kind can rattle your foundation of belief in yourself. It's understandable, but did you know everything last time? Did you know about pesticides and additives? Did you stock your fridge with fruit and vegetables that were supposed to make you drop weight like it was hot? Another reason for self-doubt is that you have bad beliefs that were engraved during your childhood. Ask yourself whether your mother always told you that obesity runs in the family and you'll always be overweight. School kids are of the cruelest kind too. Did your classmates tell you that you couldn't lose weight if your life depended on it? Listen to the answers you give yourself because you need to realize that those answers belong to someone else. They aren't your words or your self-definition.

Comparing yourself to other people is another danger to ignite self-doubt. You'll only lose yourself and your confidence if you think you're not unique from every person who walks this earth. Everyone has varied disciplines, everyone has different bodies, and our bodies all work differently. The fourth reason for self-doubt is that you're faced with a new challenge, and it's the brain's natural reaction to doubt itself. Feelings of uncertainty tend to stir discomfort. That's okay because it will drive your acceptance of the challenge. Finally, your fear of failure or success is what also makes you doubt yourself. Fear will always be built upon the first four reasons for why you doubt yourself. Don't allow past mistakes to measure future expectations.

Don't let other people's voices define you. Don't compare your beautiful uniqueness to anyone else's, and don't give way to the discomfort you feel from uncertainty. What you don't succeed at is merely a lesson to make you succeed next time. The five spokes of the self-doubt wheel flow into each other, creating a cycle that has no end and no beginning. You'll get stuck in this cycle if you don't do something about it. This is how self-doubt can stand between you and that summer body you wish you had. A lack of confidence in yourself will show physically because your mental state always reflects through your body.

Learning About Cause and Effect

Finding a diet program or lifestyle change that works for you is the easy part of this journey. Changing your mindset so that you love your body, believe in your abilities, and stop doubting your choices is the hard part. Without a mindset change, you'll be stuck in the never-ending cycle of self-doubt that loves going hand-in-hand with crash dieting and weight gain. Everything in life has a cause and effect. Think of a baby learning to walk. They have to keep trying, and yes, they fall all the time. However, practicing their little steps long enough is how they turn their wobble into a stride. It's not always about wanting to lose weight for physical purposes. It's deeper than that.

You want to eat healthier, lose weight, and live until you're sitting in a rocking chair on your porch. You want to play catch with your grandkids, and you want to fit into a bikini when you visit the beach again. This is all great, and they can all act as causes. Your mindset is the cause of this equation. Your desire to eat healthier is what motivates you and pushes you past those self-doubts. However, there are also causes working against you. Never blame yourself for cheating on your healthy lifestyle when you return from work to eat cake after a long day. The cause and effect of your entire lifestyle are constantly influencing the choices you make. It's constantly turning your self-doubt on and off.

Someone who arrives home from work and follows clean eating habits the whole day skips the drinks after work with friends, and feels good about themselves is still capable of making a mistake. Their stomachs growl and they crave sugar at night. The reason this happens, and the reason why many people give in to these cravings, is thanks to cause and effect (ShirlinaFit, 2019). Lifestyle choices during the day can also cause problems because everything leads to an effect. Maybe you're not sleeping well because being tired at the end of the day will cause cravings and hunger. You can't only look at the food you eat. Your daily habits, including sleep and everything that causes the effect of overeating, should be adjusted or you'll feel like a failure for no valid reason.

Shifting Your Mindset for Optimal Results

Changing your mindset before losing weight is the way you prevent self-doubt and lessen the chance of possible failure.

Change the Way You See Food

Stop thinking about how food makes you gain weight, the wrong types of foods, and what you can't have. Start looking at the foods that you can eat and how they can nourish the body and mind for guaranteed success. Learn to focus on the positive side of food and not the negative side. Keep telling yourself how whole natural foods are replenishing the body and making it's engine purr smoothly with nutrients. Only think about your new eating habits and how they help you to lose weight and obtain the goals you've set. You want a bikini body, you want curves that draw attention, and mostly, you want to be the definition of healthy inside and out. Your new lifestyle is a positive mindset, and you want to stay away from negative thoughts that make you doubt yourself.

Stop Negative Self-Talk

Speaking badly about yourself out loud isn't making your mindset change any easier. Don't even condone self-deprecating humor anymore. It's easy to make jokes about your need to lose weight. It's simple to undermine yourself as though you're the poster child for obesity. Your conscious mind listens to everything you say and this sets your truth. If you keep saying that you can't, then you won't. Your truth will become what you continue to joke about. Your weight isn't a joke. Self-deprecation must be forgotten. Be mindful of the words you use to describe your body.

Ground the Negative Inner Voice

Learn to live in the present. There's no judgment, rush, or need to live in tomorrow or yesterday. Keep bringing your mind back to the present with mindful practices, such as meditation, self-reflection, and experiencing every activity with your five senses. You can also make a list of counter-arguments for the times the negative voice creeps up on you again. So, your schoolmates used to tease you about the extra weight you carried. Counter this with something like: "My present habits and lifestyle changes will guarantee a body that makes them drop their jaws in time."

Talk to yourself when you self-reflect in the mirror. Don't focus on your flaws. Rather, focus on what you'll become. You can also ground yourself by having some default activities planned for the days you feel uncertain. Adult coloring, a gratitude jar, and a photo album with happy memories can bring you back to the present. Just be sure to experience every activity in full through all five senses if possible.

Stop Comparing Your Uniqueness to Someone Else

I don't care how beautiful you think another woman is. Stop comparing yourself to her. Stop comparing your abs to another man, and stop saying that your butt would look great if it was shaped like the women at the gym. Beauty isn't defined as a general rule. Everyone has a different taste. The world would be as bland as hell if everyone was defined in the same way. Also, stop looking at these models online and in movies. You don't know what time they had to arrive to reach the picture-perfect state they're in. They're wearing more makeup than what you find at Sephora. Your uniqueness is your identity and you can't be confident in yourself if you aren't comfortable with your body. Comparing yourself to "beautiful people" is the same as beating your brain with a hammer.

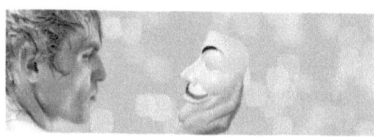

Expose Your Unique Identity

Your brain will submit to your truth again because you've taught it that you must look like skinny models to be happy. Happiness doesn't mean skinny, and you don't know what problems lie under the surface. Maybe that person is skinny because they're bulimic or have a chronic illness like Grave's disease. Your situation is different from theirs. Your desires are different and your results will be too. Comparing yourself to other people will make you focus on what you lack and this is a negative mindset. Rather look at healthy people and admire their efforts to remain so. Use them as inspiration, but don't aim to have every curve they do.

Your expectations are unrealistic if you want to look like a Playboy bunny. Remove yourself from the media that makes you feel less beautiful than models. When you first start this journey, it's best to keep your eyes off all the models in magazines and on Instagram. Comparisons aren't allowed in a healthy positive mindset. You shouldn't feed yourself with these images while your mind is still self-critical. Only follow inspiring people on Instagram that promote healthy eating and weight loss. Follow their journey and use it for inspiration.

Own Your Image From the Start

There's nothing more powerful than tricking the mind into

believing that you've already arrived at your destination. Use visualization if you must, but start showing your mind what you'd look like when you're done. Don't focus on what you look like now. Just keep feeding it your goal of what you want to look like. Let that be the only thing your mind consumes frequently.

The 21-Day Confidence Boost

Boosting your confidence can also be achieved with a simple 21-day challenge. This is a written challenge that also brings your mind back to the present reality, helps you overcome doubt, and reminds you of what you've already achieved. You can write down fears, things you're grateful for, and small achievements, and this will always be available when you feel self-doubt come back.

Day One to Seven: Write three things you're grateful for daily. You might be grateful that you lost a pound over the last few days. You could be grateful for anything whether it's big or small, because this helps you see all the things you once overlooked. You can learn how many things you have to be grateful for when you review this at the end of the week.

Day Eight to Fourteen: Now, write down the times you felt unsure and the reason why each day. This sounds negative because you shouldn't be focusing on anything but positive changes, but this exercise exposes your biggest fears and what triggers them. You can start thinking of ideas about how you'll overcome these fears in the final week.

Day Fifteen to Twenty-One: Write down the methods you used to overcome the fears daily. Don't forget to be descriptive and write your feelings down too. You feel weak when you sit in the lunchroom, looking at everyone eating their muffins and drinking soda. You decided to change this at the end of week two by sitting elsewhere. You even managed to find someone else to sit with.

The 21-day challenge boosts your confidence by making you see how you can change things. It also shows you what you have, focusing on the positive side before delving into the reasons for your lack of confidence.

Self-doubt and negative mindsets have no place in your life anymore. Once you've mastered the art of a healthy mindset, you can move on to learn more about the changes you'll make now.

STEP TWO: UNDERSTAND YOUR BODY WITH THE RIGHT TESTS

Chapter 3

Before you solve a problem, you must know what the problem is. There are a few specialty tests you can have done by functional medicine practitioners or nutritional therapists. These tests will show the levels of certain toxins within your body that holds you back from weight loss and ultimately from better health. Working with these specialist practitioners will help you design the right weight loss program that works long-term and doesn't make you slip backward.

Why Test?

The human body is a wonderfully complex design. Your immune system is responsible for protecting the body from external or foreign agents that could harm it. For example, if you twist your ankle, there's pain and inflammation that follows. This is an acute response from the immune system signaled by the brain to fix and repair the site. Inflammatory chemicals rush to the site and this allows the immune system to repair the joint. However, some people suffer from chronic inflammation and pain. The inflammation continues to thrive in the region because the immune system fails to stop it.

Too much of a good thing really is bad in this case. Chronic inflammation even causes irritating or undying pain. The immune system is capable of switching on and forgetting how to switch off. This overreaction from the immune system can also be triggered by deformed cells or pathogens in the body. Sometimes, the cells aren't always damaged, but the immune system attacks them anyway. Fatty liver cells can also be targeted as foreign agents. Fatty liver cells, scar tissue, or toxins flowing through the body are all foreign agents that activate the immune response.

Chronic inflammation caused by an overactive immune system can lead to metabolic syndrome, preventing weight loss (Esposito & Giugliano, 2004). Toxins are causing the inflammatory response, and this can also lead to insulin resistance, high triglycerides, hypertension, obesity, and low-density lipoproteins (LDL), also known as bad cholesterol. Your body can't function correctly without you removing toxic waste from your system. Toxins are found in everything you can imagine. It's in the food we eat and even the cleaning products we're exposed to.

For weight loss, we'll focus on the foods you eat and how the toxins in them can set your immune system into a self-destruct mode, making weight loss impossible and putting you at risk for multiple disorders. Bad cholesterol is to blame for heart disease and insulin resistance won't make it easy to lose weight. Besides, chronic inflammation caused by toxins can also slow your metabolism down to a screeching halt and how do you expect to lose weight then? These specialty tests have been conducted by functional medicine practitioners in laboratories. The results will help you learn what you need to avoid in your nutrition.

Functional Tests to Consider

Testing for Food Sensitivities

Being sensitive to certain foods means that the immune system responds to them. It can even overreact completely when you look at people who are highly allergic to shellfish. Their faces swell up like something from nightmares and put their lives are at risk. However, food sensitivity testing will check for every type of allergy, sensitivity, and intolerance because not everyone responds like the shellfish guy. Food sensitivity testing is great for finding foods that your immune system reacts to subtly because even low-level chronic inflammation can stand in your way of losing weight.

Being allergic and being sensitive to certain products is the same thing. The immune system still activates inflammatory agents to protect the tissue surrounding the toxin or the food ingredient your stomach dislikes. The test doesn't require more than a prick on your arm, and the practitioner will expose your tiny wound to the substance of the suspected sensitivity. This will be followed by a blood test to measure your response to the substance. Please opt for the immunoglobulin E (IgE) measurement rather than the immunoglobulin G (IgG) level because the former one is the most reliable. Your IgE levels will rise substantially when your immune system attacks exposed sensitivities.

Adrenal Fatigue Testing

Adrenal fatigue is a touchy subject as many traditional doctors refuse to acknowledge it. There isn't a specific test for adrenal fatigue, but the symptoms and responses that happen during the condition indicate that we can test for it with a stress hormone test. The adrenal glands above the kidneys are small, but they pack a powerful punch of disruptive hormones when the immune system overreacts to threats. They release adrenaline, cortisol, and dehydroepiandrosterone (DHEA). These hormones keep you alert and ready for defense against potential threats. Your heart starts beating rapidly, your blood pressure rises, and your breathing becomes fast and shallow.

Anxious people often suffer from these hormones working overtime, but being in this state too long is another damaging effect of the immune system (Philp, 2019). Having too many of these stress hormones flooding through your system can lead to heart and blood pressure problems. Stress is good for you in small controlled amounts, but being stressed all the time is just another negative response from the immune system and the brain. However, it also prevents your weight loss because the body is in constant flux against "repair and protect" signals that cause unnecessary inflammation. That's why you can use stress hormone tests to determine whether you have adrenal fatigue. Eventually, the adrenal glands become overused and shut down.

During the excessive overreaction of stress hormones, you'll suffer from mood disorders, sleep problems, and a lack of energy, which doesn't make losing weight any easier. Sleep and energy are required to lose weight, but the immune system is under attack when these stress hormones are too high. These hormones will perceive everything as threats, even when they shouldn't be. They'll start attacking normal cells and placing you at a higher risk of infections when the immune system waivers under them. The stress hormone test will determine if you suffer from adrenal fatigue. The two best options are the urine and saliva tests. There are iris contractions and blood tests as well, but your stress hormones can't be measured throughout the day unless you live in a lab.

The urine test can be used first thing in the morning, much like a pregnancy test. It will measure your cortisol awakening response (CAR) because your stress hormones shouldn't be high at this time of the day. You can then test another four to five times within twenty-four hours to make sure your stress hormones fluctuate normally and aren't high at various times of the day. Both saliva and urine tests will measure all three major hormones, and you just need to take it to your functional medicine practitioner. They'll translate the results for you and tell you if your stress hormones are causing immune system imbalances in the body because you'll have to work on this if you plan to lose weight.

Testing the Neurotransmitters

Neurotransmitters are the chemical messengers between the brain and every organ, gland, and cell in your body. They travel along billions of synapses that connect one nerve ending to another. Testing the brain's source of instructions is a surefire way to see if anything is imbalanced in the brain itself. Many neurotransmitters assist in keeping your body functioning at peak value. Some of these messengers will also aid weight loss. For example, your dopamine could be too low or high. This is problematic because it is a pleasure drug that comes naturally after achieving something you set out to do. So, you aren't experiencing the feel-good chemical when you drop five pounds. How can you feel proud of yourself if you don't experience it?

Dopamine also keeps the digestive, immune, and endocrine systems in balance. The last one is the very system where the brain and gut communicate with each other. Gut bacteria collect nutrients and send them along the endocrine system, influencing the way the brain feels. The brain also sends chemicals along the endocrine system to signal the release of chemicals in the body. Breaking this communication is detrimental and possible with too low a dose of dopamine.

Serotonin is another neurotransmitter that protects the synapses in this communications network. However, this one also regulates your body temperature, metabolism, and sleep cycles. You need good sleep and a fast metabolism to lose weight. Irregular body temperature will also keep you away from sleep. Serotonin is one of the most important chemicals in the brain. It keeps your gut healthy, and it maintains the functions of many organs. Imbalanced amounts of serotonin will result in mood disorders, carbohydrate cravings, and blood pressure issues.

Norepinephrine is another neurotransmitter that protects the synapses and it synthesizes into adrenaline. Norepinephrine regulates gut health and moods. High levels of adrenaline cause weight gain, elevated glucose levels, and problems with your attention.

Gamma-aminobutyric acid (GABA) is also a chemical messenger responsible for moods, sleep cycles, and the regulation of adrenaline. Low levels can cause a lack of energy, while high levels can make you sleepless.

Glutamate also regulates moods, calcium, and sodium levels. High levels can cause cellular damage and degenerative disorders, but high levels can keep you awake at night and mess with your adrenaline levels.

Histamine is a large player in the immune system, but it's a neurotransmitter. It keeps your gastrointestinal (GI) tract, sleep cycles, and immune system from entering unbalanced waters. Having too much histamine causes inflammation and having too little can make it hard for you to digest food.

Finally, creatinine is the last neurotransmitter that's expelled through your urine. This is what they test during the neurotransmitter testing because it cannot be influenced by other chemicals, but it shows the levels of every chemical that matters. This simple urine test determines the balance of your hormones and neurotransmitters. Imbalances will expose adrenal fatigue, mood disorders, digestive problems, metabolic syndrome, and insomnia. It's a good test to check everything you need to know about. Let your practitioner help you understand the results.

Testing Through Genetic Mapping

How better to look for genetic problems than to test your deoxyribonucleic acid (DNA) through a blood sample? This will help you determine whether you have any genetic reasons why your immune system overreacts or why you're battling to lose weight. You might also have a genetic predisposition to diabetes or insulin resistance. You might even be predisposed to conditions like polycystic ovary syndrome (PCOS), making it really difficult to combat weight loss without nutritional assistance from a licensed therapist. Looking for genetic flaws in your DNA is the best way to expose abnormal cells and manage your lifestyle and weight loss so that you don't fall into the trap of diabetes.

Genetic mapping will require a blood sample where the chromosomes, molecules, or proteins in the blood are put under the microscope. The molecular test will determine if you have any abnormalities in your single-strand DNA that should be a concern. The chromosomal test will examine the long strands of DNA to look for copies of any abnormalities and foreign cells. Remember that your body will eventually fight these abnormalities, and you won't have much success in weight loss or overall health if you don't lead a life where the abnormalities can't mutate. A practitioner will give you advice on how you can prevent genetic disorders from becoming a reality.

Testing for Environmental Toxins

Environmental toxins include the glyphosate sprayed over your wheat, but it also includes gluten which is an ingredient multiplied by these pesticides. Gluten leads to food sensitivities that cause inflammation and immune system malfunctions. It's found in non-organic wheat products like bread and flour. Natural amounts are safe for most people, but high levels of gluten can cause the body to become intolerant and your immune system will fight it. Gluten is bad, but environmental toxin testing looks for more than gluten and glyphosate.

The wheat urine test will determine whether you have an excessive number of antibodies against the wheat compounds in your system, meaning how much your immune system is responding to the wheat ingredients and residue. Your functional practitioner can tell you whether your gut is susceptible to the harmful side effects of these compounds.

You can also opt for the gut wall test that determines how strong and healthy the gut lining is. A practitioner will analyze your gut integrity with a stool sample. This test looks at the myriad of gut bacteria that make up the microbiome. If the gut is healthy, your immune system, metabolic system, and digestive system will be ready for weight loss. It's the most comprehensive test to see how the gut's health is doing.

Knowing what your test results are will help you design a personalized weight loss plan that prevents immune system malfunctions. Your metabolism needs to work at its finest. Testing all the factors and toxins that influence it is the way to maintain your weight loss.

STEP THREE: ADDING NUTRITION AND FOOD STRATEGIES

Chapter 4

Dieting is a concept that you must erase from your thoughts and your vocabulary. It's not part of what you're about to do and it has all the wrong ideas behind it. The only way you can lose weight and keep it off permanently is to slowly start changing your lifestyle and nutritional habits. You must start eating clean because being healthy and maintaining a good weight all starts with a lifelong dream. Clean eating is the way you keep those pounds away and keep the bikini or muscle body you want. To top this idea, it isn't as boring, strict, or painful as diets are.

What Does Clean Eating Mean?

Clean eating and dieting are as far from each other as you can imagine. You aren't counting calories, starving yourself, or depriving yourself of eating what you love. Registered and licensed dietician nutritionist Emily Brown, explains what clean eating is and isn't. Firstly, clean eating has nothing to do with weighing your foods and ingredients. It has nothing to do with measuring your waist and sending your weight to a dietician every week (Brown, 2016). It contains no shakes, enhancers, and liquid diets. It has no restrictions on what you can cook. It doesn't make life boring or painful. Clean eating is nothing like dieting, especially crash dieting.

Clean eating is where you make a conscious decision to change the way you see food. You live by a few rules that don't restrict your recipes or lifestyle unless you choose to be stricter for a short period. Clean eating is when you consume food that hasn't been processed to something unfathomable or sprayed with enough chemicals to cover every acre of ground in the United States (US) with eight pounds of pesticides. However, your food still contains its natural form. Food must always be nearest to its original state. You want food that doesn't contain a long list of ingredients people couldn't care to read.

You don't want food that's been modified and chemically adjusted. Clean eating encumbers whole, natural, and organic meat, vegetables, fruits, wheat, grains, oats, and healthy fats. It still has carbs, but not the kind that makes you sleepless or overweight. Refined sugars, packaged foods, and excessively processed snacks like wasabi walnuts are avoided. Everything you eat comes straight from the cow that grazes on the pasture. It comes from the harvest that contained no modifications to make the apples brighter, shinier, and tastier.

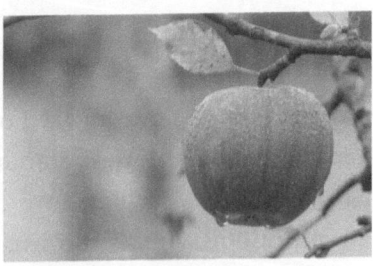

Natural Apples

In short, a meal could contain quinoa, avocado, mango, sliced apple, pumpkin seeds, walnuts, and grilled chicken on top of a bed of fresh, organic spinach leaves. There's nothing black and white about clean eating. It's as flexible as your current diet. Clean eating also doesn't mean that every carrot must be eaten raw either. Cooking, pasteurizing, steaming, and grilling foods in healthy fats are allowed. There are even amazing sweet recipes you can try by making everything from scratch with organic products. Cocoa powder is organic, and so is a cream cheese that comes from grass-fed cows.

How to Eat Clean

Allow the rules of clean eating to guide you and you won't need diets again.

Commit to Change

The first rule is as simple as committing to a long-term change in your life unless you want to return to the crash diets. Losing weight and keeping it off isn't an overnight wonder. It takes time, and you need to promise yourself that you're in this for the rest of your life.

Set Your Intentions

Knowing why you want to drop pounds, burn fat, and keep it off is how you stay motivated. Don't start this journey because your friend makes jokes about your weight. The reason why you're starting the journey should come from within yourself. Do you want to lose weight? Is it your goal or are you trying to please everyone else? The right intention will lead to the correct results. Habits can only be changed if you desire it.

Test the Waters

Starting on a lifelong journey to better health and slender bodies requires you to be open-minded and not too hard on yourself. Be willing to test the waters. Try different methods of losing weight the right way and don't beat yourself up if you fail with one. Clean eating is a journey of experimentation, and you'll feel doubt creep back in when you're too hard on yourself. Even when you make a mistake, pick yourself up and try again. Try something different to ensure that you're giving this lifelong promise the right dedication.

Slow and Steady

Ripping the bandaid off all at once isn't the best option. Take it slow and start removing certain habits that you can manage today. Then, remove one more thing tomorrow. Thanks to this being a lifelong journey, you have time to go from eating processed and chemicalized food every day to cutting back as you're comfortable. Just commit to cutting back at least one thing daily.

Healthy Eating is Unique for Everyone

Your body and context of life are unique to the world around you. Your tastes and preferences will also differ from your friends, family, and the skinny woman eating in the lunchroom. Don't expect your clean plate of food to resemble anyone else's. You might stick to using superfood vegetables, such as kale, spinach, and collard greens, but she might work better with the high-protein diet where she eats steak or eggs. Being experimental will help you design a unique food plan for yourself.

Become a Home Chef

Being experimental also allows you to concoct the craziest meals at home, but you can only do this if you're cooking. Try to cook more often than you don't. Home-cooked meals also come with the advantage of knowing precisely what goes into your food. Even a restaurant salad doesn't guarantee anything because the dressing is commercialized and processed. Have some fun with home cooking. You can start with simpler, healthy meals if you're not as used to cooking. Eventually, you might be able to reach restaurant quality standards.

Forget About Counting Calories

Counting calories is a mental block called the "diet mentality" that stands between you and clean eating. Forget about calories and focus on making food that's wholesome, tasty, and surprising. Quality will always win the mental battle because you're bound to slip up if you keep feeding yourself calorie counters, like raw carrot sticks dipped in olive oil. Most meals must taste as good as your previous experiences. Make food creative to avoid associating new eating habits with deprivation.

Use Clean, Seasonal Tricks

Nature provides you with easy recipes because what grows together also tastes great together. Experiment with same-season vegetables because they always complement each other well. Would you think that brussels sprouts and grapes taste well together? Well, try it and let me know. Squash and cranberries taste amazing together too. Nature will give us what we need. We must simply use our curious creativity to make something tasty from it. Moreover, in-season vegetables, herbs, and fruits contain higher amounts of nutrients and taste better than when they're out of season.

Keep Easy-Access Recipes

Sometimes, surfing the internet on a hungry stomach can be fruitless. Go onto websites like www.dietdoctor.com and download at least five recipes you can try for breakfast, lunch, and dinner. It's hard to be experimental from day one, but have a few recipes to try out, and start recreating them as you learn about new ingredients that add more flavor.

Read Your Labels

Unless you read the long list of ingredients, additives, enhancers, chemicals, refined sugars, trans fats, and hidden carbs, you won't know what you're consuming. Read every label and make sure it contains no more than five ingredients. Single-ingredient labels mean that the product is 100% organic, but five ingredients are fine as long as you can read and pronounce them easily. Feel free to Google the ingredients in the middle of the supermarket aisle too. No rule says you can't do this.

Burn the Processed Foods

Any highly-processed foods must be burned to the ground. Slightly-processed food is hard to avoid, such as churned, organic butter, organic or alternative milk, packaged fruits and vegetables, and whole-grain steel cut oats in a pack. The only processing you want is mechanical. Avoid chemically processed foods at all costs. So, stay away from sausages that have been turned into 30% meat and avoid canned or bottled foods. Making your foods from scratch is the better option to avoid any potential chemicals. Use fresh tomatoes instead of canned options. Use homemade salad dressing instead of store-bought dressing.

Avoid any foods with carnauba wax and soy lecithin on the labels. Try to source your food ingredients straight from the farm. Overly processed food has another name—Frankenfoods. They're grown, processed, harvested, or designed in a factory or laboratory. They contain so much salt, sugar, and trans fats that you can't lose weight while eating them. These ingredients will only play ball with your hormones and set everything off track again. Your foods should look like they would if you picked them straight from the tree. Don't fall for shiny, tasty, and artificially colored produce. Rather, eat an apple with all its flaws because nature intended it so.

The worst consequence of Frankenfoods is that they bombard your taste buds, killing them and making you less likely to appreciate the natural flavors of food. Don't worry, your pallet will restore itself and natural flavors will come back to you.

Stay Away From the Sales Pitch

Artificial flavors are there to make you want one product above another. Stay away from any product that doesn't share their "secret recipe" with you on the label. Secret recipes are a foundation of ill-health and obesity. Companies make your brain bypass the logical side and these recipes trigger feel-good chemicals to make them addictive. Suddenly, you want more and more. This also means that you should start drinking more water and avoiding all the aspartame sodas. The safest artificial sweetener is Stevia drops. Leave the sodas behind, especially the diet sodas. Beware of non-fat foods too. They also contain a vast number of artificial secrets.

Practice Makes Perfect

Practice your meal prepping to make your life simpler. Many people are deterred from clean eating because it requires more time in the kitchen. Start prepping your meals and cook enough for two or more portions at once. You can always eat the Monday-night leftovers on Wednesday night to keep it interesting as well.

Stock Up on Clean Options

Keep your pantry and freezer filled with easy and healthy options. Buy lots of fruit and vegetables. Veggies can be blanched quickly when you get back from the store and then frozen. Nevertheless, having options on hand will counter the hunger munchies you suffer from after a long day at work. Make fruit salads to stand in the fridge overnight. Buy organic yogurts and prep some healthy snacks to keep in your fridge for immediate access.

Don't Ignore Your Hunger

Your body is designed to preserve you, and the brain will send signals of hunger if you skip meals and ignore hunger cues. The longer you ignore a hunger cue, the more urgent it becomes. Always eat when hunger creeps up on you.

Remove Temptations

Humans are prone to temptation, so don't surround yourself with friends who don't support your efforts and choices. Don't have lunch with a friend daily who tries to convince you to eat unhealthily. This doesn't mean that you can't spend time with them. Just keep your temptations to a minimum.

Switch Your Carbs

Dedicate yourself to eating complex carbs instead of the refined, simple choices that break down quickly and leave you wanting more. Complex carbs take longer to dissolve and this gives you an energy boost for longer periods. Complex carbs can also promote better sleep and keep cravings at bay (Back to Health, 2020). Complex carbs are the superfood vegetables such as kale and spinach. It's also found in raw nuts, steel-cut oats, gluten-free and whole flour, and quinoa. Don't eliminate carbs totally, simply switch to eating complex carbs three times daily to sleep better and you'll have the energy needed throughout the day.

Eat Ethical Meat Products

Always buy organic meats, free-range eggs, and chickens that roam the fields. Don't buy chickens pumped full of grains to make them fall over in thirty days or less. Avoid cattle that grow up in factories eating grains instead of natural grass. You certainly don't want to see the conditions these animals must live in, never mind the steroids and chemicals injected into them for faster growth. All animal products including fish, beef, lamb, pork, chicken, turkey, eggs, dairy products, and even milk must come straight from organic and ethically-raised animals.

Beware the Fats You Eat

You've learned about hydrogenated fats that turn into trans

fats. Replace the sunflower oil, vegetable oil, margarine, and corn oils in your home with healthier options. Use moderate amounts of extra virgin olive oil, unsalted butter, coconut oil, and avocado oil. Healthy fats are also in omega-3-rich fish like salmon and mackerel. Raw nuts, seeds, and avocado also contain good fats. The natural fat in organic meat is also a source of omega-3.

Stay Hydrated

Water is the best source of hydration. Refrain from alcohol, sugary juices, and sodas as much as you can. Aim to drink eight to ten glasses of water daily. Water helps you digest food better and it keeps the brain hydrated so that your hormones remain balanced. Regulating your social temptations will also help you prevent the drinks binge every day after work. Alcohol isn't your friend because it keeps the liver busy when the liver must prioritize the toxins from booze instead of processing your nutrients and vitamins intake.

These twenty clean eating guidelines will help your weight loss, maintain it, and prevent health problems.

STEP FOUR: MASTERING THE HABIT OF BEING FIT

Chapter 5

Getting your blood flowing, hormones balanced, and your weight under control is as simple as implementing short and easy workouts into your day. These workouts don't take much time and use no equipment, but they still produce results. Exercising before breakfast in the morning can stimulate your body to burn more calories naturally because it already enters the fat-burning stage before you eat. Without wasting time, let's see what options you have to supplement your health and weight loss.

The 30-Day Challenge

Committing thirty days of being active and helping your body to burn calories isn't as insurmountable as it seems. The time and duration for your workout will depend on you. You can even implement short bursts of exercises during television commercials or in-between packing lunch for kids and feeding them breakfast. It's up to you how much time you assert at once. I'd always aim for ten-minute vigorous exercise routines during the day. Any exercise is better than nothing at all.

So, you can drop and give yourself twenty push-ups while an advertisement plays, interrupting your unmissable series at night. There's no excuse to avoid exercise. Design a 30-day challenge that suits you. Your workouts should change daily or combine multiple types of stretches, lunges, push-ups, and climbs. Changing things up daily will help the routine avoid boredom and prevent roadblocks. Choose seven different routines and repeat the routines each week. Some ideas include mountain climbing, push-ups, and cycling.

Climbing a Mountain

This sounds like you need a mountain, but fear not, you don't. The first week of your routine can include ten mountain climbs daily while you work towards thirty daily. Use a staircase or a flat floor and press on the balls of your feet while supporting yourself on your hands. Then, you can mimic the movements of a mountain climber against the floor. Bring your knees closer to your torso and feel the full cardio workout while you climb against the floor.

Bicycle Crunching

Bicycle crunches are a great workout for your abs, obliques, and hips. Lie flat on your back and place your hands behind your head. Bend your knees slightly and crunch your body. You want your left elbow to get as close to your right knee as possible, followed by the right elbow touching the left knee. Try to aim for twenty of these daily.

Planking

Planking is fun and quick, but it burns the stomach region. This sounds easier than it is, but aim for sixty-second planks daily. Rest your upper body on your forearms against the floor and raise your lower body onto the balls of your feet. Now, straighten your spine as though your life depends on it. Your entire body must be as erect as a plank.

Push-Ups

Make your push-ups exciting by changing them daily. Do five today and ten tomorrow. Also, there are a myriad of ways to do them. For the diamond push-up, you'll face the floor and move your feet so that you can press yourself up on the balls of your feet. Place both arms in a triangle position where your hands are beneath your chin, and form a diamond shape with your index fingers and thumbs touching each other. Push yourself away from the floor. The diamond push-up is a little more strenuous than the traditional type, so stick to what makes you comfortable.

Jumping Squats

This one is fun, especially if you have kids. They'll be laughing and you'll be working those triceps, calves, and buttocks. Stand with your legs shoulder-width apart and straighten your arms next to your sides. Bend your knees gently and allow the shoulders to come forward as you extend your arms in front of you. Release the position and jump when you reach the top. The biggest challenge with the jumping squats is that you'll struggle with balance at first, but aim for twenty daily.

Cycling

Cycling is a great cardiovascular workout that gives the entire body a flex. Cycling for ten minutes daily can be part of your 30-day challenge.

Mix and match your workouts to create something exciting and involve your kids if they find it fun.

10-Minute Workouts

Chances are that you want specific workouts if you're trying to lose weight and tone down precise areas of your body. There are two ten-minute options you can use for specific areas.

Beginner's Choice

This one works wonders for starting the exercise journey, and it can be implemented into the 30-day challenge. You'll be working your abs. Please note that every rest period will be ten seconds long; every exercise movement will continue for thirty seconds.

Lie flat on your back and bend your knees while you support your head in the palms of your hands. Do a middle crunch by raising your shoulders.

Rest...

Turn onto your left side and bend your knees into the same position you used for the middle crunch. Move your shoulders forward with your hands behind your head. Your torso and left elbow should be moving towards your highest knee.

Rest...

Turn to the right and bend your knees into the same position. You're going to crunch to the right now by bringing your right elbow as close to the top knee as possible.

Rest...

Lie on your back with your knees bent. Do heel touches by alternating the hand that touches as close to the heels of your feet as possible.

Rest...

Straighten your legs and raise them as high as you can while your arms are held straight against your sides, and hold your position.

Rest...

Sit with your knees gently bent and hold your hands

together in your lap. The heels of your feet must touch the ground. Now, lean backward gently and twist your hands to the left and right.

Rest...

Go back into the seated position with your shoulders leaning backward and your knees slightly bent. Cross your arms over your chest and maintain this hold.

Rest...

Position yourself for mountain climbing. Keep raising those knees close to your upper body, and alternating between them.

Rest...

Enter your plank position and hold it, remembering to keep your back and legs straight in a line.

Rest...

Now, lie on your back and raise your legs to the sky. Use your arms to stretch toward your feet in the toe touches exercise.

Rest...

Switch to the bicycle crunch now by bending your legs and placing your hands behind your head. Start alternating so that the right elbow touches the left knee and the left elbow touches the right knee.

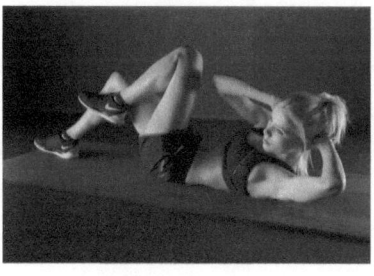

Bicycle Crunch

Rest...

To do a hip lift, you'll remain on your back and raise your legs. Use your arms for leverage and push your legs even higher. Drop them and push them up again, never losing the support of your arms. Add a swing back and forth for your legs to make it more productive.

Rest…

Go back into an ab hold by raising your legs again and stretching your arms straight along your sides while you hold this position.

Rest…

Now, use the spider plank by supporting yourself on your hands and the balls of your feet. Run your left foot along your calf to make a triangle and then you can run it back down. Alternate to the right leg and do the same.

Rest…

End your ten-minute ab workout with another plank. Keep those legs straight with your back and support yourself with your forearms.

You're all done with the abs. Use this workout for a productive exercise routine in your 30-day fitness challenge.

Belly-Burner

This is a low-impact full-body workout that targets belly fat and the legs. You'll use thirty-second exercises with five-second breaks this time.

Go into a knee pull by scissoring your legs and facing a 45-degree angle. Raise your arms above your head and bring them down as you raise the back leg upward to meet your hands.

Rest…

Now, switch sides and do knee pulls on the opposite leg.

Rest…

Go from a side lunge into a curtsy. Stand with your hands in front of your face as though you're praying, and lean towards your left side. Your left knee must bend and support your body while your right leg is straight. When you bring the support knee back, shift your support to the right leg and allow the left leg to step behind the right one. Open your hands while you swing backward.

Rest...

Repeat the side lunge into a curtsy on your right leg now.

Rest...

Clasp your hands in front of your chest and get down on your knees. Now, using one leg at a time, get up from your knees before you use one leg at a time to go back down.

Rest...

Enter the superman plank now before you start raising your left leg and right arm to straighten them. Keep your balance and bring them back in before you alternate to the right leg and left arm.

Rest...

Enter the squat front kick by separating your legs shoulder-width and dropping down with your hands in front of you. Allow your shoulders to come forward slightly and give a kick forward when you rise again.

Rest...

Next, do the crab squat by getting into the squat position, dropping down, and alternating which leg steps forward and then backward. Rise and drop again while the other leg steps forward and backward.

Rest...

Do a traditional push-up and then stand. Step back, step forward, and then do another push-up. Keep doing this for thirty seconds.

Rest...

Go back onto the floor and get ready for mountain climbing. Remember to bring your knees as close to your upper body as possible with each step.

Rest…

Go into a side plank position by resting yourself on your left forearm and facing towards the wall. Your legs are resting on the side of your left foot. Raise your right hand over your shoulder and bring it back.

Rest…

Go into the side plank position on your right side now, and raise your left arm over your shoulder before bringing it back.

Rest…

Now, you'll do some corkscrews. Go into the push-up position and bring your left leg under your core, kicking it out to your right side while touching it with your right hand. Come back and alternate to the other leg and hand. This one requires some balance, but you'll get it.

Rest…

Next, sit on your butt and rest your upper body on your hands placed flat on the ground slightly behind you. Raise your legs and kick them forward while your upper body moves back gently.

Rest…

Go into a table position and raise your core as high as possible. Rest on your hands and feet to make a table shape. Rise and drop your core.

Rest…

Do a shoulder tap now by positioning yourself in the traditional push-up stance. Raise your left hand and tap your right shoulder before dropping it. Now, alternate to the right hand and left shoulder.

Rest…

Do reverse lunges by standing straight and scissoring your left leg backward while your right knee bends. Your hands will come up to meet in front of you, and you can bring the leg back. Alternate to the other leg and continue this lunge movement.

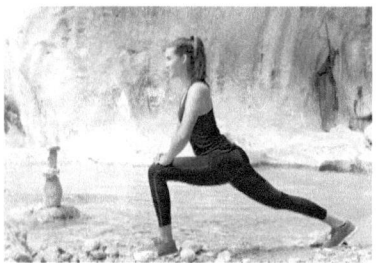

Forward Lunge

Rest and replenish yourself with some water because you've completed another ten-minute workout.

Endless Possibilities

I've shared some examples with you, but cardiovascular exercises, such as walking, cycling, and swimming also do wonders for you. Cardio gets your blood flowing better to every organ in the body, reducing backlash from potential disorders and aiding in weight loss (Lindberg & Bubnis, 2019). This protects your heart, brain, and kidneys, ensuring proper function throughout the body. Oxygen carries nutrients to the organs and this delivery system works well when your heart is pumping healthily with cardio workouts. However, 150 minutes of cardiovascular workouts are required weekly to sustain weight loss and maintenance.

This can be divided throughout the week to ensure that you have rest days too. Working out for five days would require thirty minutes daily. Cardio exercises can be achieved with a five-mile fun run, cycle, or walk. Why not divide the fun run into a triathlon of all three? Combining your cardio workouts with flexible or tension training will help you build muscles while you're losing weight. Depending on how much weight you have to drop, most people want to tone up as soon as the pounds melt away. Otherwise, they're left with loose skin and flabby arms.

Finally, you can also add meditation yoga to your routine. It helps you stretch your body into positions that open the pathways for nutrients and vitamins to reach every organ. You learn to control your breathing and posture to guide the oxygen to where it's needed. Stretching can also help you combat inflammation and tenderness in your muscles, giving them back the ability to repair themselves. Join a yoga group nearby, especially those that practice in the park. It will also teach you how to relax and see exercise through a new light. Starting a fitness routine after being overweight and sedentary is hard, so you're welcome to start with exercise twice a week until you get into the 30-day challenge.

STEP FIVE: ADDING A FEW CELLULAR CHOICES

Chapter 6

Your body will transform into a new shape and your fitness will climb the stairs of better health and lower weight, but you still need to consider a few more tactics in your weight loss journey. You've learned about clean eating, easy exercise routines, and how to test for toxins and food sensitivities that make it hard to lose weight. Now, you'll be introduced to methods you can use to enhance your weight loss journey and strip toxins from the body. Being fit and slender is one thing, but being healthy on a cellular level is another thing.

Detoxing Your Body

There are some toxins and chemicals in your body that prevent steady weight loss, and they put you at risk for additional health problems. Detoxes are optional because not every glove fits every hand. There are numerous options, such as juice cleanses, foot baths, and colon cleanses. However, there's one type of cleansing you can choose if you're ready to restore the body and give back its ability to regenerate, burn fat, and remove toxins from every corner of your body and mind. Cellular detoxes are based on five simple rules.

1. Remove the source that's causing toxins and preventing weight loss. You're already doing this when you start to eat clean.
2. Regenerate the intelligent part of your cells called the membranes. Replacing your unhealthy trans fats with healthier options can promote the regeneration of cellular membranes. The membrane is crucial because it collects nutrients and helps to regulate hormones.
3. Restore energy to the cells. The mitochondria in your cells process the nutrients and turn fat into energy. This can be restored by eating complex carbohydrates.
4. Reduce the inflammation surrounding the cells. You can avoid sugar, grains, and unhealthy fats to start the reduction. You can also introduce anti-inflammatory ingredients to your diet such as cayenne pepper, tomatoes, leafy greens, and olive oil.
5. Re-establish the natural methylation or self-healing function of the cells. Keeping your diet as clean from toxins as possible is the way to go here. You can also speak to your functional medicine practitioner about a methylation donor supplement.

These five rules will go through three stages.

1. The preparation stage is where you avoid toxins and enhance the five rules of cellular detox with a whole

diet. So, avoid those pesticides, additives, "secret recipes," and artificial flavors for thirty days.
2. The body stage comes next, and this is where you maintain the five rules, but you want to open the pathways so that your toxins can be removed from your brain in the last stage. This also lasts for thirty days and you can now add colon cleanses, kidney flushes, and coffee enemas at will. This opens all the organs that need to flush the body of toxins. You can also eat potassium-rich foods to help this stage along.
3. The final stage is called the brain phase, and it also lasts 30 days. You'll need a binding agent while you still follow the five rules. Speak to your practitioner about a binding agent that can bind and expel toxins right from the brain through the body. Some options to try are *Bind* and *CytoDetox*. Use binding agents for no longer than seven consecutive days, and then you must leave it for up to ten days.

Cellular detoxes are the deepest form you can use. They help your cells, which make up every part of your body and mind, to restore themselves so that fat-burning, weight loss, and better health are on the cards for you. It might seem long if you think of ninety days in total, but remember that your weight loss is a lifelong journey. Your better health is a lifelong goal. So, ninety days is merely a drop in the ocean.

There are some products suggested for use from stage two by holistic nutritional therapists. Add zeolites for optimal absorption of vital nutrients and minerals, and add glutathione as an antioxidant to protect the downstream cells from collecting the upstream toxins in stage three. Astaxanthin is another antioxidant that protects the cells and restores their self-healing abilities from stage two (Novak, 2020). Don't use supplements other than methylation donors in the first thirty days of your cellular detox and avoid binding agents in stage one.

Intermittent Fasting for Weight Loss

One of the new raves out there works. Intermittent fasting is when you time your meals. It isn't about starving yourself; it gives your cells the energy to restore themselves and burn fat before you replenish your calories again. Intermittent fasting has vast benefits, including the release of the human growth hormone (HGH), which turns on the fat-burning process and maintains muscle mass (Gunnars, 2018). Your body is starved of carbohydrates and calories for short periods so that the liver can release ketones to attack the fat cells and convert them to energy. The body and brain go into the autophagy stage where cells start to regenerate themselves.

Fasting will also prevent insulin spikes that stop autophagy and weight loss. Insulin only breaks your fast. Your cells will also repair themselves and remove harmful proteins and chemicals from their structure in the autophagy process. Finally, your genes will express themselves, meaning that they'll switch over to protection mode, and longevity is also sustained. In brief, intermittent fasting can help your body turn fat into the enemy because no calories and carbs are swarming around. Intermittent fasting isn't a diet either.

It's a corrective lifestyle that you implement for one or two-week stretches at a time. The best option is to follow the 16-8-hour rule. This means that you fast for sixteen hours and restore the calories your body needs for eight hours. So, you're not starving yourself at all. Start your fast at 10:00 PM and you'll be eating at 2:00 PM again. There are a few rules of successful fasting.

1. Prepare your body for the fast by eating a meal made of protein, healthy fats, and fiber at 10:00 PM.
2. Consume nothing but black coffee or tea with no creamer and sweetener for the fast period. Drink between eight and 10 glasses of water during a 24-hour cycle.
3. Stay away from alcohol for two hours after breaking your fast with food.
4. Don't use your protein shakes, pre-workout supplements, or smoothies in the fast period.
5. Don't use nutritional supplements that aren't water-soluble.
6. Break your fast at 2:00 PM with a simple bone broth that doesn't contain a combination of fats and carbs. You can either eat carbs and protein combined, or you can try fats and protein combined. Don't mix carbs and fat because they'll open your cells for insulin spikes.
7. Plan your workouts during your fast. You'll burn more fat while the body's already in this state and your muscles *won't* be affected.
8. Plan shorter fasts at first if you're a woman. Women have higher levels of estrogen, the reproductive hormone, flooding through their bodies, and it can cause an influx of hunger cravings. Women can start with a 12-hour fast period.

Intermittent fasting brings you one step closer to your weight goals, but it also helps the body and mind maintain better health.

It even increases your focus because your brain doesn't have much energy, so it needs to prioritize tasks to use what energy is available. I've designed a simple fasting guide for you. The entries are flexible, but you get a weekly idea of what can be done. Stretch it to two weeks the next time you fast. I recommend fasting every two to three months to ensure that the cells are regenerating and the autophagy process is in place. Besides, it will prevent you from gaining weight when your body learns to use fat for energy.

	Monday	Tuesday	Wednesday	Thursday	Friday	Saturday	Sunday
8:00 AM	exercise/water	exercise/water	exercise/water	water	exercise/water	exercise/water	tea
9:00 AM	water	tea	tea	water	tea	black coffee	water
10:00 AM	tea	black coffee	water	black coffee	water	water	water
11:00 AM	water	water	water	water	black coffee	tea	water
12:00 AM	water	water	water	black coffee	tea	water	black coffee
1:00 PM	black coffee	tea	tea	tea	water	black coffee	water
2:00 PM	vegetable broth	bone broth	fat/protein	complex carbs	bone broth	fat/protein	carbs/protein
3:00 PM	water	tea	water	tea	water	tea	water
4:00 PM	clean lunch	clean lunch	clean lunch	clean lunch	clean lunch	clean lunch	clean lunch
5:00 PM	tea	water	water	water	tea	water	black coffee
6:00 PM	clean dinner	clean dinner	clean dinner	clean dinner	clean dinner	clean dinner	clean dinner
7:00 PM	black coffee	water	water	water	water	black coffee	tea
8:00 PM	water	water	tea	water	water	water	water
9:00 PM	light snack	light snack	black coffee	light snack	black coffee	water	light snack
10:00 PM	fat/fiber/protein	fat/fiber/protein	fat/fiber/protein	fat/fiber/protein	fat/fiber/protein	fat/fiber/protein	fat/fiber/protein

You'll notice that you eat four to five times daily which is optional. This is merely a sample schedule. The reason why it says clean lunch and dinner is that you must never forget your clean eating rules. Where it says complex carbs, use the superfood vegetables, such as collard greens and kale. Light snacks also need to remain light because you're about to eat a large fiber meal at 10:00 PM. Your fast-breaking meals don't need to be huge either. They can be between four and six ounces. The broths allow your stomach to absorb nutrients after a fast period, so they're great options, and best of all is that you can pre-cook them.

The Keto Lifestyle

The keto lifestyle is considered a diet, but it doesn't need to be. The reason why the keto diet has turned heads is that it also activates cellular autophagy (Kubala, 2018). I'm sure you've noticed how this entire chapter is advice on how to keep your body burning fat instead of carbs. You'll turn your body into a fat-burning pound-dropping machine by the end of it. The fact remains that every inch of your body and mind are made of cells or molecules. These cells need the energy to survive, and leading a keto lifestyle gives them just that. You're replacing your carbohydrate intake which the body has used to create energy until now with healthy fats.

The number one rule of the keto diet is to consume 75% healthy fats, 20% organic protein, and only five percent carbs. The fats can't include sunflower oil, omega-6 fats, trans fats, or hydrogenated fat. It must contain natural omega-3 fats found in mackerel, salmon, herring, sardines, grass-fed beef, extra virgin olive oil, flaxseed oil, raw walnuts, chia, or flax seeds. Carbs also can't contain the regular run-of-the-mill types. They must contain complex carbs that take forever to break down. Organic, whole, and pesticide-free grains, superfood vegetables, and quinoa are some options. Proteins must also be organic and free from any chemicals, including meat, dairy, and eggs.

Your body breaks down the fat and proteins to use this for energy and restoration. You don't have to weigh your food. You simply have to live by the 75-20-5 rule. You can adjust it slightly to 70-25-5 if you prefer this. Your liver starts producing ketones, which are molecules processed through fat when glucose levels are low. This starts the ketosis process that keeps your body in the fat-burning state as long as you're avoiding anything more than five percent carbs. You'll be eating no more than around twenty to thirty grams(g) of carbs daily, or you'll stop the ketosis and need three to four days to restore it. The chart below can help you see how many carbs are in a cup of vegetables because you want most of your carbs coming from them. The carbs are measured in grams per cup.

1 Cup	Carbs	1 Cup	Carbs	1 Cup	Carbs
Spinach	1.1 g	Chard	1.3 g	Bok Choy	1.5 g
Romaine Lettuce	1.5 g	Collard Greens	2 g	Mushrooms	3.1 g
Celery	3.5 g	Cucumbers	3.8 g	Zucchini	4 g
Radishes	4.3 g	Eggplant	4.7 g	Cabbage	5 g
Asparagus	5.3 g	Cauliflower	5.7 g	Broccoli	5.8 g
Tomatoes	5.8 g	Red Bell Pepper	5.8 g	Kale	6.7 g
Green Bell Pepper	6.9 g	Spaghetti Squash	7 g	Brussel Sprouts	7.9 g
Green Beans	9.9 g	Carrots	12.3 g	Leeks	12.6 g

As you can see, vegetables contain more carbs than you think. However, this table will help you keep track of your carbs through cup portions instead of weighing everything. The table below will show you what is recommended on the keto lifestyle.

Food Types	Recommendations
Eggs	Only organic, free-range eggs are allowed
Poultry	Free-range chicken and turkey
Fatty seafood	Wild salmon, herring, and mackerel
Meat	Grass-fed beef, pork, venison, bison, and organ meats (everything must be organic)
Dairy	Full-fat cream, unsalted butter, and yogurt
Cheese	Organic and full-fat cream cheese, brie, goat's milk cheese, mozarella, and cheddar
Raw seeds and nuts	Flax seeds, sunflower seeds, macadamia nuts, walnuts, peanuts, and almonds
Natural spreads	Organic and additive-free peanut, cashew, and almond butter
Healthy oils	Extra virgin olive oil, peanut oil, coconut oil, and avocado oil
Complex carbs	See the vegetable chart above
Spices	Fresh, organic herbs, whole spices, Himalayan salt, and coarse black pepper
Condiments	Fresh lemon juice, vinegar, and balsamic vinegar

The keto lifestyle is similar to eating clean, and you don't need to weigh anything as long as you're portioning your fats as the majority of your intake and keeping your carbs to the recommended allowance. Stay away from baked goods such as bread, muffins, cookies, and cracker bread. Avoid all refined sugars and diet sodas. You want full-fat products and not fat-free additives. Stay away from pasta, white rice, cereals, nonorganic oats, and wheat. You also want to avoid starchy vegetables like potatoes, corn, peas, pumpkin, and butternut squash. Fruit must be removed from the keto diet as well because it contains too many simple carbs and natural sugars. Alcohol should also be restricted on the keto lifestyle.

This gives you one more tactic to restore and rejuvenate your cells while burning fat effortlessly.

The Value of Sleep

Sleep also restores our energy to face a new day, giving us more energy to exercise and enjoy our meals. However, sleep is much more than this when it comes to weight loss. In fact, sleep deprivation increases your chance of obesity and sustained weight problems by 89% (Pullen, 2017). Losing sleep can make you gain weight because your body produces more of the hunger-stirring ghrelin hormone and less of the leptin hormones that make you feel full. Sleep can improve the way your brain works, regulating the neurotransmitters during the day, keeping your appetite at bay.

Everyone cycles through non-rapid-eye movement (non-REM) and rapid-eye-movement (REM) stages of sleep every ninety minutes. Your body temperature drops and the brain signals restoration and regeneration during the non-REM stages. The REM stage is where you dream, and this happens because your memories are being consolidated. However, it's the restorative stage that matters because your cells and muscles need to replenish themselves so that you have enough energy throughout the day. Your brain and body are so energy-deprived when you don't sleep enough that the brain starts releasing the hunger chemicals.

Your decision-making is also affected, leaving you with little to no willpower to sustain your clean eating and weight loss desires. Your brain can even become so deprived that it starts craving foods, carbs, and sugars to release feel-good chemicals in this state. Your metabolism also slows down because the body burns a lot of calories and fat from the cells while you sleep. Remember that you can teach your metabolism how fast it needs to work, so depriving it of sleep long enough will send the wrong message. Finally, you could be making your body insulin resistant with a lack of sleep. When this happens, the cells won't absorb the minor glucose intake anymore and the pancreas will overproduce insulin.

I think the value of sleep has become clear if you intend to lose weight and keep it off while keeping your cells healthy. Maintaining a good sleep schedule of eight hours per night will help you lose weight and sustain metabolic health.

STEP SIX: BREAKING AWAY FROM THE FORK IN THE ROAD... THE PLATEAU

Chapter 7

You must know that your body and mind will retaliate when you lose weight. There will be obstacles, a loss of motivation along the way, and the inevitable plateau that comes with every weight loss journey. Most people don't know what happened when they reach the fork at the crossroads and sadly they choose to go back to their previous lives because it seems like they've failed. Knowing why these forks happen, and how you can break through them is a vital part of sustaining weight loss and optimal fitness. Let's look at the most common obstacles you can expect.

Standing Your Ground

The first obstacle you'll encounter is when all motivation slips from your grasp. The sad truth is that many failed diets start with a lonesome journey. Dieting and losing weight is a long-term goal meaning that a lack of support is going to drop your motivation down the deepest pits of hell. Remember that your weight loss and desire for fitness is a personal goal; it doesn't consider what other people told you to do. It's your pursuit, but any journey that lasts this long is bound to become boring, unmotivated, and lack all excitement if you travel alone. It's time for you to recruit a wholesome support group that stands with you all the way.

You want cheerleaders rooting for every pound you drop. You need people holding you accountable for the promises you made to yourself. The moment you start eating clean, detoxing, fasting, or using any wholesome method to lose weight and gain a perfect body tone is the moment you need people supporting your efforts and acknowledging your achievements. Losing motivation is the brain's way of retaliating against weight loss. The brain hates change and wants everything to remain the same. It will push doubts into your mind, telling you that it's okay to cheat once in a while. It's okay to drop your clean habits and stop exercising for a week.

No, stand your ground and say enough is enough. *The Journal of Consulting and Clinical Psychology* published a study confirming whether you're more likely to succeed with a support group. Two groups of participants took part in the study, totaling 166 people. The first group had three friends or family members to keep tabs on them, hold them accountable, and give them support throughout their ten-month weight loss journey. The second group was consuming the same calories, exercising the same, and following all the guidelines set, but they had no support. The four-month follow up proved that having support was a true motivator.

Ninety-five percent of supported participants completed the program and 66% of them maintained their weight loss when following up at ten months. Only 76% of the unsupported participants completed the program and a minuscule 24% of them maintained weight loss over ten months (Wing & Jeffery, 1999). These figures don't lie, and you're better off with a support group. Join a local exercise group, and enlist some friends to hold you accountable. Give a family member the responsibility of your weight records weekly, and surround yourself with people who only push you forward.

Hitting the Plateau

Another reason for losing motivation and wanting to give up is when you hit the inevitable plateau that comes with weight loss. The first truth you must always remember is that you *will* hit the plateau, especially if you're losing big chunks of weight. A weight-loss plateau happens when you've been following every clean eating habit, detox, exercise routine, and keto rule, but you still hit a wall where your weight stands still, mocking you. Climbing on the scale was once an exciting exercise, but now it's mentally challenging because the needle stays in the same place.

The plateau is perfectly natural because your body is fighting against the changes. It normally happens after you've been losing weight for a few months, or you've lost a few bricks of fat already. There are a few reasons why this happens.

Weight Set-Point

Firstly, the body's set-point of weight you learned about is working against you. The set-point hasn't developed overnight and you shouldn't expect the body to accept the changes so fast either. Chances are that the set-point has developed over the years. The body and mind's first and foremost instinct is to preserve itself in homeostasis, meaning that it will halt your weight loss or slow it down to a treacle when it feels threatened. The good news is that your body and mind are flexible, but it takes time. Be patient and give the body four weeks to catch up with your new intentions. The body doesn't know that you intend to lose more weight. Give the metabolism time to readjust to the new set-point. Maintain your new lifestyle and make the necessary adjustments after the four weeks if your weight still stands.

Metabolic Pause

Your metabolism needs to readjust according to your body mass. The metabolism functions at speeds necessary to maintain the energy processing, depending on what your current weight is. So, the lower your weight, the slower the metabolism will react because it has fewer calories and fat stores to burn. Your metabolism already has a resting rate, which is the number of calories and fat molecules it burns before you eat and exercise during the day. This is also happening while you sleep. It isn't only your lifestyle and food that determines how fast your metabolism functions. It also functions while you're sleeping, burning fat cells and converting them into energy for when you wake up. It can't work at the speeds it did before because the body has fewer fat stores.

Worst of all is that your metabolism is still regulated by the primal need to preserve your body, and it will process fewer calories to sustain weight or even make you gain it again to reach the set-point. Fortunately, you can break through the metabolic response if you're patient and determined enough. Start with more strenuous exercises that build muscles because muscular metabolic cells remain more active than the fat-based cells. The keto lifestyle also helps because eating 25% protein daily will feed the muscles, keeping them active. However, the other method of jolting your weight loss to bypass the metabolic pause is to decrease your calories. Your metabolism has learned to burn fewer calories now and you can counter this by feeding it less.

Doctor Alexandra Sowa from the American Board of Obesity recommends dropping your calorie intake by 20% every time your body mass drops by 10% (Fetters, 2018). This will kick-start the metabolism to burn all the calories you eat and you won't be left with leftovers at the end of the day.

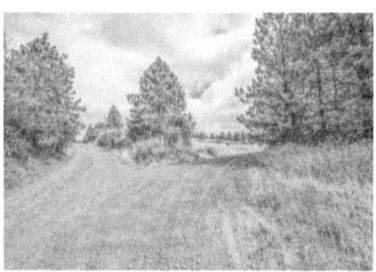

Decisive Plateau

Fitness Milestones

Think about the first time you tried squats or lunges. You felt uncoordinated, unbalanced, and shaky. Let's not forget that you felt like you were doing it wrong. The second time you squatted, you felt more confident, balanced, and coordinated. From that point, squats became more natural every time you exercised. Your body's adaptability is both a friend and an enemy on the weight loss journey if you don't know how to keep training it. Compare it to riding a bicycle to understand it better. You'll fall a bunch of times, but eventually, your legs and arms know precisely how to get the bike moving forward and how to make it defy gravity.

Your body is turning exercise into a second-nature as you grow fitter. You don't even have to think about doing it anymore because it's part of your daily routine after a few weeks or months. There's no heaving and shakiness anymore. Your focus, movements, and follow-through are as smooth as a baby's bottom. The body doesn't only adapt either. It also improves the efficiency of how you exercise with every routine. Simply, the body starts burning less and less energy with each workout. That explains the first part, but there's another truth that should be common sense. I know that common sense isn't always at the forefront when you're disappointed with the scale or mirror, but it remains.

The more fat, calories, and weight you have to burn, the harder it is to exercise, making it a fat-burning struggle to do twenty push-ups if you weigh 200 pounds. However, someone who weighs 100 pounds won't require the same effort and intensity of exercise. They'll need more challenging workouts to force the body to burn fats, tone muscles, and shape them like a model. Stagnant exercise routines can also cause a plateau of weight loss. There's a simple solution for this. Change your exercise routine every four weeks to prevent the body from getting too comfortable with them. Add more strenuous workouts with every change, and push yourself harder and longer.

Plateaus are just another hurdle you can jump over. And guess what? You'll be slimmer and fitter to do just that when they come. Never give up because of a temporary problem. Making a permanently negative decision to combat a temporary problem is like dowsing flames with gasoline. Remember to keep your mindset positive, and know that you can overcome plateaus. Thinking you can't is like giving in to the self-doubt you already overcame.

Quick Fix for Breaking the Plateau

Preparation is the master of all successful outcomes. Prepare for the plateau to ensure that it doesn't last long or knock you off your motivation track. Your memory can fail you especially if the brain desires it, but your personal track records can help you stay ahead of the game. Start with a food diary where you keep records of what you eat. You can take it as far as counting calories if this doesn't deter your dedication. Counting calories will help you drop 20% every time you lose 10% of your body fat. There are some wonderful smartphone applications you can download to keep track of your intake and your calories. Having your record at the touch of your fingers is one way to simplify your weight loss if you choose to count calories.

The first choice is *MyFitnessPal*, which is the most popular right now.

The second choice would be *Lose It*, which counts calories, diarizes your foods, and logs your exercise routines.

The third app is free and it's called *FatSecret*. It's a simple design to count calories.

I just want to remind you that healthy living with a lifelong goal of sustaining weight loss isn't always about counting calories. This is an optional choice for you to cut back when the plateau comes. The other obvious choice is to cut your portion sizes as your body needs fewer calories. This doesn't require an app. You can simply cut your portion size down as your weight drops. Don't even wait for the plateau. Lastly, track your exercise types and routines from day one so that you can change it every four weeks. Push yourself a little harder every month, especially if you're retaining weight around your belly.

Men statistically drop weight more easily than women, but they also tend to keep it around the midsection. Women expand in their legs, stomach, and even upper body, but men must always be wary that they can carry more weight around the middle, maintaining their risk for diabetes, insulin resistance, and heart problems. Anyone with midsection weight that's sticking around longer than the rest of their bodies must implement ab workouts and intensify them monthly.

You can leap over the obstacles as they come as long as you know they're coming.

STEP SEVEN: TREAT YOURSELF DESERVEDLY

Chapter 8

You're well on your way to fat freedom and erasing the plagues on your health. It might be a long journey, depending on your current weight, but it will be a fruitful one filled with rewards and pleasures. In fact, not adding the rewards will only backfire on you. You're about to learn how the reward loop works and how you can use it to sustain a clean and wholesome life where you're as fit as you choose to be.

Hijacking the Reward Loop

Nothing makes weight loss more real than watching the achievements and rewarding the milestones. Sometimes, you can easily lose sight of the outcome when the journey is too long. You lose motivation and your discipline waivers. However, it doesn't seem so insurmountable when you break the outcome into smaller journeys. It's frightening to think of losing forty pounds, but breaking it into smaller portions is how it loses its paralyzing effect. Moreover, each small step brings you one step closer to the outcome. The picture below helps you understand the importance of baby steps.

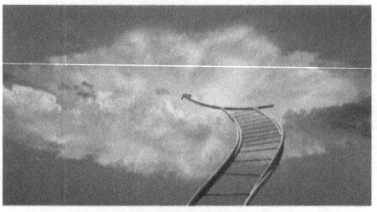

Ladder Goals

THE LADDER'S foot is where we all start when we set goals. The clouds are where we intend to be one day, but the rungs are the most important part of the ladder. Without the rungs, you can't take another step closer to the top. Spacing the rungs too far apart will work against you. You want the rungs to be close to each other to offer support, sturdiness, and constant steps. You also want them far enough apart so that each requires an individual, measurable step. Life requires balance, and so does weight loss and health. However, you need motivation before you step onto the next rung or you'll lose sight of the end of the ladder that's hiding in the clouds.

Each rung must be followed by a small reward, or you won't be motivated to reach the next one. The reward loop is the part of your brain that releases dopamine every time you accomplish something (Lee, 2017). It's a feedback loop to keep you interested in a task once you've started. Dopamine is the most powerful motivator and it comes from inside your brain. It's the same neurotransmitter that encourages cravings when the brain and synapses need comfort. It runs along the synapses and empowers them for stronger communications, and the stronger it becomes, the more likely you are to continue.

The secret to sustaining your weight loss goals and climbing every rung until you reach the clouds is to hijack your dopamine. You can control it by exercising, and showing the brain just how proud you are of the step you've just climbed. Having small goals or short rungs allows you to hijack the dopamine frequently to feed your reward loop more often. The only trick is that you need to know when you've reached a new rung.

Climbing the SMART Ladder

Your weight loss and fitness goals must be broken into small, sustainable steps, and each step must be SMART. This is an acronym that represents the rules of specific, measurable, attainable, relevant, and timely goals. Break every goal into smaller steps that follow all five rules to ensure your potential.

Specific

Being specific about each goal will help you acknowledge them when you arrive. For example, don't only say that you want to drop five pounds. Turn your stepping goal into something tangible and visual. You could say that you want to drop five pounds and visualize the precise context of this goal. Where will you be when you accomplish this? Will you be standing on your scale?

Visualize the place, clothes you're wearing, and even the denim shorts you want to fit back into. I always close my eyes and envision every aspect of my goal to be specific. Be specific about how you're going to achieve this too. Note your exercise routine, food plan, and dietary changes you'll make to achieve the five-pound drop. Don't leave anything out of your vision and take notes to make sure you can keep track of it.

Measurable

Every step on your journey must be measurable meaning

that you must know when you've arrived. Breaking your goal into smaller portions of five pounds already makes it measurable. You have a total of 20 pounds to lose, but you're sticking to five pounds per milestone.

Achievable

Are you capable of achieving the goal you set? Look at your notes and be realistic about whether you can achieve the desired outcome. It doesn't help to stumble over something unachievable before you even start because this will knock your confidence and motivation down. Losing five pounds is reasonable because you can see it when you look in the mirror. You can afford the foods you must buy, so that's also achievable. You can also attend classes.

Relevant

Give your notes one more review to see whether every milestone has relevance. You won't visualize yourself lying on the beach to drop five pounds, but your exercise routine is relevant to the goal.

Timely

Finally, give every step of your ladder a time frame. How long do you want to strive to lose five pounds and how long do you need to complete the twenty pound long-term goal? Timely means that you must set a time to start and end each goal. I'll start first thing in the morning and give myself two weeks to achieve a five-pound drop.

Keep in mind that every rule of SMART goals complements another one. So, don't be unrealistic about your start and end times because this doesn't tick the achievable box. Measurable and timely rules also go hand-in-hand, and your relevancy and likelihood of achieving your goal work together. Being specific is seen in every rule of the SMART system. Now, set some goals and keep track of your milestones because every achievement, no matter how big or small, will come with a pleasurable reward.

Rewarding Each Rung

Before you even dive into this section, know that rewards don't include daily food cheats and drinking binges. Rewards must be pleasurable, but they can't undo everything you've already achieved. Otherwise, you'll be taking one step forward and sliding five rungs down. Rewards also aren't restricted to weight shed. You could reward yourself for the first five-mile run completed or for the first three days that you completed a ten-minute workout. Set goals for your nutrition, exercise routines, and choices, and then reward them as you complete them.

You can even reward yourself for quitting smoking or you can seek pleasure after going an entire week without eating refined sugars or drinking alcohol with friends. Finally, make sure your rewards fit your finances so that you don't suffer from unwanted stress at the end of the month. Let's see how many options you have under the five types of rewards you can enjoy.

Budget Rewards

We can't all book a trip to Hawaii when we drop twenty pounds, but there are awesome budget options available. Treat yourself to any budget reward for small accomplishments. You could subscribe to a new magazine, upgrade your Netflix package, or buy a new soundtrack to exercise with. Choose music that speaks to your soul so that you enjoy it and it doubles as a motivator. You could also try a home spa day or movie night at home or the theatre. Buy yourself some flowers, a new book, or a potted plant. Why not get a new water bottle or journal? There are many ideas you can opt for that will cost you less than $10.

Adventurous Rewards

Most of us have some adventure or travel enthusiasm inside of us. These rewards, depending on your budget, can be saved for bigger achievements, or use local trips that cost less for milestone achievements. Go on a camping trip with friends, spend a day at the beach, or hike up a mountain. Larger budgets with larger achievements can look at weekend getaways and exploring new trails two towns over. Adventurous rewards don't only include travel either. Why not buy a new hiking bag, camping equipment, or upgrade your travel accessories? Buy a new camera and take it on a tour of the city. You can also look for cycling tours to double your reward as a sensory, nature adventure. Heck, jump from a plane, or visit the museum if you want to. Give yourself rewards that make you want more.

Pampering Rewards

Pampering yourself is also a budget-friendly option most of the time. Self-care is a vital part of leading a healthy lifestyle, and you aren't just losing weight, you're also looking after yourself. Get a massage, do acupuncture, or sign up for a floating session or hydrotherapy. Go to the spa for the day or join a yoga class. Keep in mind that these options are for men and women because there's nothing wrong with a man that cares for himself. Buy some aromatherapy candles or essential oils to make your home resemble a spa. Self-care rewards can also be found in self-improvement and self-help books. Buy a new one and implement what makes you feel better.

Random Reward Explosion

The ideas standing in plain sight are endless too. Whatever makes you feel happy is what you should reward yourself with. Go for a manicure or pedicure. Why not do both? Buy yourself some new workout clothes and strut your stuff. You'll need new outfits and workout clothes as the pounds drop anyway. Add new sneakers and buy some home equipment when you're ready. Low-cost home gym equipment includes resistance bands, yoga mats, and foam rollers. Color your hair or get a tattoo. Have a girl's or boy's night out and allow yourself a minor cheat once in a blue moon. A glass of dry red wine or moderate tequila has the fewest calories in them. Otherwise, have a slice of cheesecake every month or so.

Attend a concert or buy yourself a Fitbit or Apple watch to keep track of your fitness enhancements. Hire a personal trainer or sign up at the gym. Splurge some money for new headphones because they're great for workouts too. Sign up at the local escape room with a group of friends or take lessons in something you've always wanted to try. Feeding your hobbies are also a great reward. Learn to play an instrument or take lessons for scuba-diving, pottery, surfing, or skiing. Pay for a session with a functional practitioner and upgrade your meal plan. Buy your favorite perfume, cooking classes, or a new cookbook that fits the clean eating lifestyle. Purchase a bicycle and start a new exercise routine.

Mindful Rewards

This one might be a little challenging at first, but getting comfortable and closing your eyes to visualize the journey you've completed can also reward the brain. Revisit the moment you stepped on the scale and all the sensory aspects of how you felt at that moment. Rekindle the time you completed your first five-mile run and how it made you feel. Immerse yourself with all five of your senses when you visualize your accomplishments so that you can teach your brain to remember how the experience made you feel.

Rewards are the final part of losing weight and keeping it off. Let's face it, you deserve a reward after shedding pounds or running a marathon. Even small changes deserve rewards. Now, you have everything you need to become slender, fit, and maintain optimal health.

AFTERWORD

The world might fade, the diets might be at war with each other, the statistics might speak for the majority, but you will shine. The days of breathless heaving, sweating through your favorite shirt, and covering up every love handle are gone. Obesity and weight problems are common, and so are the fad diets that rage through our lives. Drink this tea daily, pop this miracle pill to lose fifty pounds, and eat endless smoothies to shape yourself. I know you're just as tired of seeing these blatant lies as I am.

Being overweight is a hard life that comes with many consequences. You're prone to develop diabetes, blood pressure problems, and mood disorders. Happiness escapes the reality in front of you when you're bombarded with advice that doesn't even work. Everyone expects you to drop those pounds like someone who donates blood at the blood bank. Heck, wouldn't that be amazing if we could all afford to suck it out? Life is, unfortunately, a little harder than that when the pounds pile on.

It makes you feel like you have no energy left. Fat cells strip you of the life you deserve, and who cares? The media doesn't care because they just want to sell their lies to you. The food industry certainly doesn't care either. You care, and that's all that matters. You want to live life to the fullest, be fit enough to enjoy your kids, go on adventures with friends, and be able to strut your amazing body anywhere. You want to turn heads, and you're sick of using all these empty promises to do it.

If only there was a way to lose weight the same way you gained it. In this book, you've learned exactly how to do that. You know that every tiny habit you change is working towards a larger picture. The myth of restricting everything you love eating was blown to shreds. The fallacy that you need to make drastic and enormous changes are hammered to the ground. You don't need to believe the lies anymore because you get to choose your weight, how you implement the changes, and when you see the results.

You know what harm the fad diets are doing to your body. You've learned about the toxic products hidden in plain sight. Nothing is standing in your way of putting one foot ahead of the other at a time. You won't get a better idea of what's going on in your body than what the five weight loss preparation tests can show you. Your mindset has changed for the better, and even this happens slowly. Pounds don't latch onto you overnight, and you can't change everything you know at once to correct your weight.

You know what you need to eat now and the rules to follow, so throwing away the foods you love isn't necessary. Eating clean is the way to lose weight without losing your creative edge either. You have exercises that help you tone specific parts of your body and burn fat from other parts. Who knew it could be as quick as ten minutes daily? Ten minutes is nothing compared to the benefits you'll achieve. Moreover, you'll have

Afterword

four foundational techniques to reset your body so that weight problems never haunt you again.

You can remove what you don't want from your system, use cellular secrets to restore the body to its natural form, and you'll enjoy the rest you deserve. Overcoming the inevitable obstacles can't be easier than what you've learned, and it requires little to no effort from your side. Learning how to control the reward loop in your brain is how you make sure that every small step forward counts. This yo-yo mentality won't affect you again because you know how to fuel the fire of the most straightforward habit changes.

The best news is that you don't need to apply everything at once. Go easy on yourself and experience the pleasures that come from being slender, toned, and healthy. I've enjoyed guiding you along with the only lifestyle change you'll ever need. I'm passionate about natural transformation because human biology wasn't designed for the many existing bad options on the market. Besides, we don't all have thousands of dollars to spend on weight loss. You have everything your new life needs, and now you can take that first step, however shaky it might seem at first.

Slow down and focus on you, your journey, and what your desires need. Feel free to share your successful journey through the seven minor habit changes you've implemented to make a big splash in the pool of accomplishment. Reach out to me in the reviews and let others know how your journey has helped you. I'm rooting for you, and so are your cheerleaders you've set up. You can do this, and you'll be reaching for the stars in no time. Go and be the person you've always desired because only you can write your conclusion.

Plee From Author

Hey Reader, you got to the end of my book. I hope this means you enjoyed it. Whether or not you did, I would like to thank you for giving me your valuable time to try to entertain you and you found valuable content that was helpful. I'm truly blessed I can have this opportunity, but I only have this opportunity because of people like you; people kind enough to give my books a chance and spend their hard-earned money buying them. For that I'm entirely grateful.

If you would like to find out more about my other books then please visit my website for full details. You can find it at:
www.amazingjaqproducts.com/publishing

Also feel free to come and join our Facebook Group as I would love to have you be part of our growing community that is eager to stay healthy.

If you enjoyed this book and would like to help, then you could think about leaving a review on Amazon or anywhere else that readers visit.

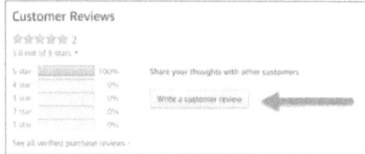

I have posted below the link directly to Amazon as it is always a challenge how to find it on Amazon. The most important part of how a book sells is by how many positive reviews it has, so leave one and you are directly helping me to continue my journey as a full-time author and publisher. Thanks in advance to anyone who does. It means alot!

www.amazon.com/review/review-create/asin=

REFERENCES

Back to Health. (n.d.). *Testing*. Back to Health Natural Solutions. https://www.backtohealthnaturalsolutions.com/testing/

Back to Health. (2019a, October 11). *How to stop having pain all over*. Back to Health Natural Solutions. https://www.backtohealthnaturalsolutions.com/how-to-stop-having-pain-all-over/

Back to Health. (2020, September 28). *Eat the right carbs and sleep better*. Back to Health Natural Solutions. https://www.backtohealthnaturalsolutions.com/eat-the-right-carbs-and-sleep-better/

Ben, K. (2016). *Changing your mindset for weight loss | self love & body image*. YouTube. https://www.youtube.com/watch?v=sQQv8EoKi4U

Brown, E. (2016). *What does it mean to eat clean?* Mayo Clinic. https://www.mayoclinic.org/healthy-lifestyle/nutrition-and-healthy-eating/in-depth/what-does-it-mean-to-eat-clean/art-20270125

Chui, A. (2017, March 23). *How self doubt keeps you stuck (and *how to overcome it)*. Lifehack. https://www.lifehack.org/567587/the-reasons-of-self-doubt-and-steps-to-deal-with-it

Cleveland Clinic. (2019b, October 1). *Why people diet, lose weight and gain it all back*. Health Essentials from Cleveland Clinic. https://health.clevelandclinic.org/why-people-diet-lose-weight-and-gain-it-all-back/

Delicious, C. (2017). *A beginners guide to healthy eating | how to eat healthy | 15 tips*. YouTube. https://www.youtube.com/watch?v=jwWpTAXu-Sg

Drah, H. (2020, January 7). *26 Most disturbing weight loss statistics*. Loud Cloud Health. https://loudcloudhealth.com/resources/weight-loss-statistics/

Empowered Health. (2018). *True cellular detox*. Empowered To Heal. https://www.empoweredtoheal.com/true-cellular-detox

Esposito, K., & Giugliano, D. (2004). The metabolic syndrome and inflammation: Association or causation? *Nutrition, Metabolism, and Cardiovascular Diseases: NMCD*, 14(5), 228–232. https://doi.org/10.1016/s0939-4753(04)80048-6

Fetters, A. K. (2018). *3 reasons you've hit a weight-loss plateau – and how to break through*. US News & World Report. https://health.usnews.com/wellness/food/articles/2018-02-09/3-reasons-youve-hit-a-weight-loss-plateau-and-how-to-break-through

Gunnars, K. (2018). *Intermittent fasting 101 — the ultimate beginner's guide*. Healthline. https://www.healthline.com/nutrition/intermittent-fasting-guide

Kubala, J. (2018, August 21). *A keto diet meal plan and menu that can transform your body*. Healthline. https://www.healthline.com/nutrition/keto-diet-meal-plan-and-menu

Lee, K. (2017, September 22). *The science of motivation: Your brain on dopamine*. I Done This Blog. http://blog.idonethis.com/the-science-of-motivation-your-brain-on-dopamine/

Lindberg, S., & Bubnis, D. (2019, May 8). *How much cardio do I need to lose weight? Here's what works*. Healthline. https://www.healthline.com/health/how-much-cardio-to-lose-weight

Living Young. (n.d.-b). *Pesticides and processed foods rob the body of nutrients*. Living Young. https://livingyoungcenter.com/pesticides-and-processed-foods-rob-the-body-of-nutrients/

MadFit. (2019). *10 min cardio workout at home (equipment free)*. YouTube. https://www.youtube.com/watch?v=sjmsApWcyCU

Matthew, N. (2020, March 11). *30 day workout challenge to get fit in 2020*. Talk District. https://www.talkdistrict.com/30-day-workout-challenge-to-get-fit-in-2020/?utm_source=bing&utm_medium=cpc&utm_campaign=US%20Campaigns&utm_term=30%20day%20exercise%20challenge&utm_content=30%20Day%20Workout%20Challenge%20To%20Get%20Fit%20In%202020

Medline Plus. (n.d.-c). *What is genetic testing?: MedlinePlus genetics*. Medline Plus. https://medlineplus.gov/genetics/understanding/testing/genetictesting/

Neurogistics. (n.d.-d). *Neurotransmitter testing*. Neurogistics. https://www.neurogistics.com/products/neurotransmitter-testing#:~:text=A%20neurotransmitter%20test%20provides%20information

Novak, S. (2020, January 9). *This 5-step expert-backed guide will detox your body down to the cellular level - organic authority*. Organic Authority. https://www.organicauthority.com/energetic-health/expert-guide-detox-body-cellular-level

Pal, M. (n.d.). *3 pieces of weight loss advice for men*. Self Growth. https://www.selfgrowth.com/articles/3-pieces-of-weight-loss-advice-for-men#:~:text=You%E2%80%99re%20going%20to%20plateau.%20This%20is%20usually%20the

Philp, T. (2019, July 18). *Adrenal fatigue and stress testing - complete guide (2019)*. Healthpath. https://healthpath.com/adrenal/adrenal-fatigue-test-guide-2019/

Pullen, C. (2017, June 6). *7 ways sleep can help you lose weight.* Healthline. https://www.healthline.com/nutrition/sleep-and-weight-loss

Raman, R. (2017, October 29). *Is it bad to lose weight too quickly?* Healthline. https://www.healthline.com/nutrition/losing-weight-too-fast#TOC_TITLE_HDR_3

Reif, P. (2020). *10 min beginner ab workout / no equipment.* YouTube. https://www.youtube.com/watch?v=1f8yoFFdkcY

ShirlinaFIT. (2019). *CAUSE & EFFECT - weight loss motivation & mindset | workout motivation.* YouTube. https://www.youtube.com/watch?v=2iyxClnjzHo

Sorey, K., & Sorey, K. (2020, February 12). *50+ non food weight loss rewards & goals reward chart.* Sorey Fitness by Kim and Kalee. https://soreyfitness.com/fitness/50-weight-loss-rewards/

Ting, C. (2020). *10 min morning routine to burn belly fat | no jumping.* YouTube. https://www.youtube.com/watch?v=xyR8McQnGuw

Wing, R. R., & Jeffery, R. W. (1999). Benefits of recruiting participants with friends and increasing social support for weight loss and maintenance. *Journal of Consulting and Clinical Psychology,* 67(1), 132–138. https://doi.org/10.1037/0022-006x.67.1.132

Image References

Bicycle Crunch. (n.d.). Pixabay. https://pixabay.com/photos/sport-training-abdominals-sixpack-2250970/

Decisive Plateau. (n.d.). Pixabay. https://pixabay.com/photos/fork-road-dirt-direction-path-two-2115485/

Expose Your Unique Identity. (n.d.). Pixabay. https://pixabay.com/photos/man-view-mask-self-knowledge-4008575/

Forward lunge. (n.d.). Pixabay. https://pixabay.com/photos/young-woman-girl-sporty-nature-2699780/

Ladder Goals. (n.d.). Pixabay. https://pixabay.com/photos/heart-head-beyond-clouds-sky-2748340/

Natural Apples. (n.d.). Pixabay. https://pixabay.com/photos/apple-fall-juicy-food-autumn-1122537/

Slow and Steady. (n.d.). Pixabay. https://pixabay.com/photos/road-sign-asphalt-road-sign-90390/

www.ingramcontent.com/pod-product-compliance
Lightning Source LLC
Chambersburg PA
CBHW021128080526
44587CB00012B/1189